DEFIANT CHILDREN
Second Edition

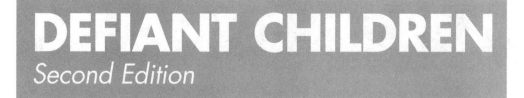

DEFIANT CHILDREN
Second Edition

A Clinician's Manual
for Assessment and Parent Training

RUSSELL A. BARKLEY, PhD

THE GUILFORD PRESS
New York London

Once more, for my parents, with love and gratitude,
Mildred M. Barkley
and Donald S. Barkley

And in loving memory of my stepmother,
Rebecca Mercer Barkley

© 1997 The Guilford Press
A Division of Guilford Publications, Inc.
72 Spring Street, New York, NY 10012

Printed in the United States of America

This book is printed on acid-free paper.

Last digit is print number: 9   8   7   6   5   4   3   2

Library of Congress Cataloging-in-Publication Data

Barkley, Russell A., 1949–
    Defiant children : a clinician's manual for assessment and parent
training / Russell A. Barkley. — 2nd ed.
      p. cm.
    Includes bibliographical references and index.
    ISBN 1-57230-123-6
    1. Behavior disorders in children.   2. Behavior therapy for
children.   3. Child rearing.   4. Parent and child.   I. Title.
    [DNLM: 1. Parenting. 2. Behavior Therapy—in infancy & childhood.
3. Child Behavior Disorders—therapy.   HQ 755.7 B256d 1997]
RJ506.B44B36   1997
618.92'89—dc21
DNLM/DLC
for Library of Congress   96-47746
                                          CIP

Preface

This manual, as was the first edition, is an effort to set forth the sequence of procedures for training parents in child management skills that I have employed during the past 20 years of my clinical practice, and that, in large measure, is the culmination of over 30 years of research and clinical experience by others. For the past 15 years, I have taught these procedures to over 6,000 mental health professionals in the United States and Canada as part of a series of 1-day workshops. The response to these workshops has been most gratifying. The majority of those attending not only found these procedures to be extremely useful in their clinical practice with families, but also encouraged me to develop a manual of these techniques, which could serve as a clinical handbook for wider dissemination to child mental health workers. I am genuinely grateful to these individuals for this encouragement, as it led to the first edition of this book. Similar encouragement more recently has resulted in my revision of the original manual. This revision has permitted me to (1) increase dramatically the references to the scientific literature supporting the rationale for the program and efficacy of its procedures, (2) expand the number of assessment tools provided herein and bring the original assessment materials up to date, (3) revise the instructions for carrying out the original steps of the program based on additional research and clinical experience, and (4) create an additional training session for parents on how they can assist with improving their children's school behavior.

The roots of this parent training program began in a set of methods developed by Constance Hanf, PhD, Professor Emeritus at the University of Oregon Health Sciences Center, more than 25 years ago. The program, referred to as a "two-stage program" for child noncompliance, consisted at that time of two fundamental procedures designed to teach parents more effective ways of dealing with child noncompliance. Parents were first taught an effective method of attending positively to ongoing appropriate child behaviors, particularly compliance with requests, while ignoring inappropriate behavior. After this, parents were instructed in a second procedure consisting of the immediate use of time out following child noncompliance with a command. In combination, these procedures proved to be a powerful treatment package for parents dealing with noncompliance in their children. Practice of the methods in the clinic under therapist supervision was an essential part of this program, as was the use of simply worded, brief handouts on the use of the methods at home. Many psychology interns and fellows, including myself, were blessed with the opportunity to acquire these skills during our training at that institution with Dr. Hanf, as the procedures had not been published or widely disseminated. Those wishing to read more extensively about the original program can refer to the text by Forehand and McMahon (1981) for the details of the procedures, as well as to the extensive research Dr. Forehand and his colleagues and students conducted in the 10 years prior to that publication.

During the past 20 years of using this program, I have had occasion to expand and modify it to deal with populations of children with Attention-Deficit/Hyperactivity Disorder, Oppositional Defiant and Conduct Disorders, or more serious behavioral disturbances. An introductory session has been added to Hanf's original program to explain more fully to parents the development of misbehavior, and especially noncompliance, in children. More details are also provided on teaching parents not only to reinforce direct compliance with requests, but also to encourage children to play independently of their parents when the parents cannot be interrupted. The inclusion of a variation of the Home Chip Program (Christopherson, Barnard, & Barnard, 1981), in a modified form, to Hanf's original program was necessitated by the realization that seriously and chronically behavior disordered children are not as consistently responsive to social praise and affection as are normal children. Hence, a more powerful means of reinforcing child behavior was needed to increase and sustain child compliance with parental requests. Sessions have also been added to Hanf's original program so as to address specific problems in dealing with noncompliant child behavior in public places (stores, restaurants, etc.) and in preparing parents to manage future misbehavior that may arise with the child. Despite these changes, I have tried to remain true to the principles of the original program, including the requirements of homework assignments for the parents and the use of brief, simply worded parent handouts to augment the training occurring in the treatment sessions.

The program described here owes much to the stimulating, heuristic, and collaborative discussions I have had over the years with others trained in the original program with whom I have been fortunate to associate. Charles Cunningham, Eric Mash, and Eric Ward have been the most instrumental in my modification of the program and formulation of new components for it based on current research and clinical practice. I am also grateful to Arthur Anastopoulos, George DuPaul, Terri Shelton, Mariellen Fischer, and Gwenyth Edwards for their comments and suggestions for improving this training program. The writings of and my discussions with Rex Forehand, Robert McMahon, and the faculty at the Child Development and Rehabilitation Center, Oregon Health Sciences University, have also made significant contributions to this program.

I am indebted to Peter Wengert for his encouragement of the first edition of this manual and to Seymour Weingarten and Robert Matloff of The Guilford Press for their encouragement of this second edition and their support for all of my writing efforts. I continue to express my sincere gratitude to my wife, Pat, and children, Stephen and Kenneth, who unselfishly gave of their family time so that this project might be completed. The wisdom I have gained from the unique experiences with my own children is undoubtedly woven into the fabric of ideas expressed here. Finally, I owe a great deal to the more than 1,200 families of behavior problem children to whom I have had the fortunate experience to teach this program. Many of their suggestions for improving this program are contained herein.

RUSSELL A. BARKLEY, Ph.D.
Worcester, Massachusetts

Contents

Introduction   1

Part I   Prerequisite Information for Using the Program   15

Chapter 1   The Rationale for the Program   17
Chapter 2   Clinical Assessment of Defiant Children   44
Chapter 3   Practical Considerations in Parent Training   73
Chapter 4   An Overview of the Parent Training Program   81

Part II   Guidelines for Therapists in Conducting Each Step   89
              of the Program

Step 1   Why Children Misbehave   91
Step 2   Pay Attention!   102
Step 3   Increasing Compliance and Independent Play   111
Step 4   When Praise Is Not Enough: Poker Chips and Points   120
Step 5   Time Out! and Other Disciplinary Methods   131
Step 6   Extending Time Out to Other Misbehavior   145
Step 7   Anticipating Problems: Managing Children in Public Places   147
Step 8   Improving School Behavior from Home: 155
              The Daily School Behavior Report Card
Step 9   Handling Future Behavior Problems   159
Step 10   Booster Session and Follow-Up Meetings   162

Part III Assessment Materials   165

    General Instructions for Completing the Questionnaires (Form 1)   169

    Child and Family Information Form (Form 2)   170

    Developmental and Medical History Form (Form 3)   171

    Disruptive Behavior Disorders Rating Scale—Parent Form (Form 4)   174

    Disruptive Behavior Disorders Rating Scale—Teacher Form (Form 5)   176

    Home Situations Questionnaire (Form 6)   177

    School Situations Questionnaire (Form 7)   178

    How to Prepare for Your Child's Evaluation (Form 8)   179

    Clinical Interview—Parent Report Form (Form 9)   188

    Adult Behavior Rating Scale—Self-Report of Current Behavior (Form 10)   213

    Adult Behavior Rating Scale—Self-Report of Childhood Behavior (Form 11) 214

Part VI Parent Handouts for Steps 1–10   215

    Parent Handout for Step 1: Profiles of Child and Parent Characteristics   219

    Parent Handout for Step 1: Family Problems Inventory   220

    Parent Handout for Step 2: Paying Attention to Your Child's
        Good Play Behavior   222

    Parent Handout for Step 3: Paying Attention to Your Child's Compliance   225

    Parent Handout for Step 3: Giving Effective Commands   227

    Parent Handout for Step 3: Attending to Independent Play   228

    Parent Handout for Step 4: The Home Poker Chip/Point System   230

    Parent Handout for Step 5: Time Out!   233

    Parent Handout for Step 7: Anticipating Problems—Managing Children
        in Public Places   237

    Parent Handout for Step 8: Using a Daily School Behavior Report Card   240

    Parent Handout for Step 9: Managing Future Behavior Problems   247

References   248

Index   262

Introduction

Purposes of the Program

This manual is designed to serve several purposes. First, it sets forth detailed instructions for conducting clinical evaluations of defiant or behavior problem children. In so doing, a set of interview forms and behavior rating scales that may be employed by clinicians for conducting such evaluations is also provided. These may be photocopied, as necessary, with some limitations (see the copyright page for details). Some forms are also designed to be used for the periodic evaluation of the parent's and child's responses to the treatment program throughout training and shortly after its completion (posttreatment evaluation). Second, and more to the point, this manual specifies the step-by-step procedures to follow in conducting a highly effective, empirically validated program for the clinical training of parents in the management of behavior problem children. Careful attention was paid to preparing the format for the presentation of each step of the program so that the manual would be of utmost practical use in conducting the training program, including using a comb binding for the manual so that it can lie flat on a desk or clipboard for easy reference during training sessions with parents. And third, this manual provides a set of parent handouts to be used during the course of the program. These handouts include forms to be completed by the parent as well as instructions to the parent for use with each session of the program. The handouts are designed to be easy to read and to be brief in content. They are not meant to be used, however, in isolation from training by a skilled child/family therapist.

Understand that this manual and the program it describes are not intended for use by individuals who have not had education and training in the knowledge and skills necessary to provide mental health services to behavior problem children and their families. Professionals using this program should have adequate training in child development, child psychopathology, social learning and behavior modification techniques, and other clinical interventions with families as may be required. In short, this program is not a substitute for either general clinical training or the careful exercise of clinical judgment and ethics in dealing with behavior problem children and their families. The utmost care is always required in tailoring these methods to the individual characteristics of a particular child and his/her family.

This manual is also not intended to be a review of the scientific literature on parent training programs or research on behavior problem children. Satisfactory reviews of this literature as well as other, similar approaches to parent training have been published in numerous forums (see Dangel & Polster, 1984; Forehand & McMahon, 1981; Mash & Barkley, 1989, in press; Mash, Hamerlynck, & Handy, 1976; Mash, Handy, & Hamerlynck, 1976; Patterson, 1982; Patterson, Reid, & Dishion, 1992; Patterson, Reid, Jones, & Conger, 1975; Wells & Forehand, 1985). The reader may wish to consult these and other sources for conducting parent training programs (Schaefer & Briesmeister, 1989) before undertaking this particular approach. The manual instead is intended to be a clinical handbook for conducting only those procedures pertinent to this particular sequence of child behavior management methods.

Types of Children Appropriate for This Program

As with any clinical procedure, this program was not designed as a blanket method to be applied to all children regardless of their presenting problems or the concerns of their families. It is expressly intended for children who display noncompliant, defiant, oppositional, stubborn, or socially hostile behavior alone or in conjunction with other childhood disorders. These children are often referred to as having "externalizing" or "acting out" disorders and may go under the more generic layman's labels of difficult, defiant, or aggressive children, or the more specific clinical diagnoses of Oppositional Defiant Disorder (ODD), Attention-Deficit/Hyperactivity Disorder (ADHD), Conduct Disorder (CD), atypical Pervasive Developmental Disorder, or even juvenile-onset Bipolar Disorder, provided that noncompliant or defiant behavior is a primary problem with the children. The program is also quite applicable to children with mild developmental delay (mental retardation) where child noncompliance or defiance is a problem for parents. Despite being intended for use with clinically referred populations of children, however, portions of the program also may be quite valuable for use with mild situational behavior problems in otherwise normal children whose families are being seen for more general parent, marital, or family therapy. In particular, children displaying difficult, "acting out," or defiant behaviors as part of adjustment reactions to parental separation or divorce often respond well to the methods in this program. In short, where children exhibit problems with listening to and complying with parental commands or requests, or with adhering to household or neighborhood rules, this program will prove quite useful.

The program was designed for children having a language or general cognitive developmental level that is at least at a 2-year level and having a chronological age that falls between 2 and 12 years. Although it is possible to use the program with children as young as 18 months of age, the success of the program greatly hinges on the child's level of receptive language development in that the child must have the capacity to comprehend parental commands, directives, and instructions. Children below age 2 years with delayed language development will respond less successfully to this program, or their families will require greater training time and practice than families of children without such delays. Also, some parts of the program (except time out) may be used with children 13 years of age or older, depending on their level of social maturity and the severity of their behavior problems. Immature preadolescents with mild to moderate noncompliant behavior can be successfully treated with this program with appropriate modifications accounting for their greater level of mental development and their desire to be autonomous and to participate in the family's decision-making process concerning their behavior. For children older than 13 years of age, however, I recommend the behavioral family therapy program designed by Arthur Robin (1979, 1981, 1984) with Sharon Foster (Robin & Foster, 1989) or the similar program of Forgatch and Patterson (1987). Those programs concentrate more heavily on teaching family problem-solving, communication, and conflict resolution skills than does the present parent training program.

The present program has been successfully employed with single-parent as well as two-parent families, those of low income or educational levels, or even abusive families, although again the constraints noted above apply here as well. Even where the child in an abusive family is not defiant, this program can serve to provide parents with more humane and effective methods of dealing with the everyday management of such a child.

Whereas the program can certainly stand alone, and often does, as the primary form of intervention provided to parents of defiant children, it can also serve as an adjunct to other forms of therapy being provided to troubled parents or families who also happen to have misbehaving children. Many therapists have found a behavioral parent training program to be highly useful as an adjunct to marital counseling, when disagreements over child management are an issue in the marriage (see Sanders, 1996, for a discussion), or to psychotherapy with anxious, depressed, or otherwise maladjusted adults who are also having problems managing the behavior of their children. The program can also serve as part of a larger treatment package for socially aggressive, oppositional, or conduct problem children, who may themselves benefit from the addition of direct child training in social problem-solving skills (Kazdin, Esveldt-Dawson, French, & Unis, 1987; Kazdin, Siegel, & Bass, 1992).

Goals of This Program

The present program has a limited number of goals but is highly effective at accomplishing them with most families. These are as follows:

1. To improve parental management skills and competence in dealing with child behavior problems, particularly noncompliant or defiant behavior.

2. To increase parental knowledge of the causes of childhood defiant behavior and the principles and concepts underlying the social learning of such behavior.

3. To improve child compliance with commands, directives, and rules given by the parents.

4. To increase family harmony through the improvement of parental use of positive attention and other consequences with their children; the provision of clear guidance, rules, and instruction to those children; the application of swift, fair, and just discipline for inappropriate child behavior; and general reliance on principle-guided parenting behavior.

Outcomes Expected from This Program

The procedures described here have a substantial amount of research supporting their efficacy (Anastopoulos, Shelton, DuPaul, & Guevremont, 1993; Forehand & McMahon, 1981; McMahon & Forehand, 1984; Patterson, 1982; Patterson, Dishion, & Chamberlain, 1993; Patterson et al., 1992; Sanders, 1996; Webster-Stratton, 1982; Webster-Stratton & Spitzer, 1996). Each procedure is supported by published studies demonstrating significant improvements in child behavior as a function of these or highly similar behavior management methods being adopted by parents, including (1) *improving parental selective-attending skills* (Eyberg & Robinson, 1982; Forehand & McMahon, 1981; Kelley, Embry, & Baer, 1979; Patterson, 1982; Pollard, Ward, & Barkley, 1983; Pisterman et al., 1989; Roberts, 1985; Webster-Stratton, Hollinsworth, & Kolpacoff, 1989), (2) *improving parental deliverance of commands* (Blum, Williams, Friman, & Christophersen, 1995; Forehand & McMahon, 1981; Green, Forehand, & McMahon, 1979; Patterson, 1982; Roberts, McMahon, Forehand, & Humphreys, 1978; Williams & Forehand, 1984), (3) *improving children's solitary play behavior* (Anastopoulos et al., 1993; Pollard et al., 1983; Wahler & Fox, 1980), (4) *parental use of time out* (Anastopoulos et al., 1993; Bean & Roberts, 1981; Day & Roberts, 1982; Eyberg & Robinson, 1982; Forehand & McMahon, 1981; Patterson, 1982; Pisterman et al., 1989; Roberts, Hatzenbuehler, & Bean, 1981; Roberts et al., 1978; Strayhorn & Weidman, 1989; Wahler & Fox, 1980; Webster-Stratton et al., 1989) and (5) *response cost as disciplinary methods* (Anastopoulos et al., 1993; Little & Kelley, 1989), as well as (6) *parental planning and activity scheduling as problem prevention measures,* particularly before entering public places (Anastopoulos et al., 1993; Pisterman et al., 1989; Sanders & Christensen, 1984; Sanders & Dadds, 1982; Sanders & Glynn, 1981).

However, the degree of success is greatly affected by the extent, nature, and severity of the child's psychopathology and that of the family, among other factors (see "Predictors of Success and Failure," below). With children whose major problem is noncompliance or oppositional behavior and whose families are not seriously dysfunctional, this program usually results in bringing the child's behavior and compliance within the range considered normal for children of that age group. In my experience, children with more serious forms of developmental psychopathology, such as ADHD, ODD, CD, or atypical Pervasive Developmental Disorder, that are chronic in nature may be improved in their compliance under this program (Anastopoulos et al., 1993; Johnston, 1992). Nevertheless, after treatment, many may continue to be rated as more deviant in inattentive and impulsive behavior than normal children on child behavior rating scales, particularly if the children had significant degrees of symptoms of ADHD before treatment (Anastopoulos et al., 1993; Johnston, 1992). With such children, the attitude taken is one of training parents to "cope" with the child's problems rather than "cure" them; yet the program can minimize the extent to which child noncompliance contributes to the child's various problems and the distress within the family.

Children older than 12 years of age or those who are seriously aggressive and assaultive with others should not be considered candidates for this program. They often do not respond or their reaction to the procedures results in an escalation of family conflicts. In rare instances, there may be an increase in the adolescent's already destructive, verbally aggressive, or even physically assaultive behavior, creating even more distress for the family than existed prior to treatment (Barkley, Guevremont, Anastopoulos, & Fletcher, 1992). Older children have had more years of effectively utilizing coercive behavior (especially that involving physical as well as verbal resistance), are more severe in the degree of defiant and conduct problems, may have more frank psychiatric disturbance, and may come from more disrupted or impaired families (Dishion & Patterson, 1992; Patterson et al., 1992). For all of these reasons, then, older children may benefit less from parent training programs, although benefits may still accrue to some older children and their families (Barkley, Guevremont, et al., 1992; Dishion & Patterson, 1992). Severely aggressive and defiant older children and adolescents may be better treated with multiple and more intensive in-clinic therapies (Patterson et al., 1993), with in-home multisystemic forms of therapy (Mann, Borduin, Henggeler, & Blaske, 1990), or within treatment foster care, day hospital programs, residential treatment facilities, or inpatient child psychiatry units, at the conclusion of which parents can be trained in this program to prepare them for the children's return to the home.

Parents with at least a high school education who have minimal degrees of personal or family distress are likely to do quite well in acquiring and utilizing the skills and knowledge taught in this program. These parents are also more likely to report high levels of consumer satisfaction with the training procedures (Calvert & McMahon, 1987; Forehand & McMahon, 1981; McMahon & Forehand, 1984; Patterson, 1982; Sanders, 1996; Webster-Stratton & Spitzer, 1996). The methods taught in this program have received high levels of acceptability when reviewed by other adults or by the parents who are the direct recipients of training (Calvert & McMahon, 1987; Kazdin, 1980; McMahon, Tiedemann, Forehand, & Griest, 1984; Sanders, 1996; Webster-Stratton & Spitzer, 1996). Such parents report not only improved child behavior (Anastopoulos et al., 1993; Bernal, Klinnert, & Schultz, 1980; Dubey, O'Leary, & Kaufman, 1983; Eyberg & Robinson, 1982; Forehand & McMahon, 1981; Patterson, Chamberlain, & Reid, 1982; Pisterman et al., 1989; Pollard et al., 1983), but also demonstrate changes in directly observed parental behavior (Patterson, 1982; Patterson et al., 1982) and better attitudes toward their children (Forehand & McMahon, 1981; McMahon & Forehand, 1984; Webster-Stratton et al., 1989). Parents trained in child behavior management skills also reported increased knowledge of parenting skills, reduced parenting stress, and an improved sense of self-esteem and parenting competence (Anastopoulos et al., 1993; Pisterman et al., 1989; Spaccarelli, Cotler,

& Penman, 1992; Spitzer & Webster-Stratton, 1991); better sibling behavior (Eyberg & Robinson, 1982; Humphreys, Forehand, McMahon, & Roberts, 1978); and better marital and family functioning (Forehand & McMahon, 1981).

Maintenance of Treatment Gains over Time

A number of studies have examined the extent to which parents and children continue to manifest improved interactions with each other once treatment has been terminated. Improvement in child behavior, parent behavior, and parental attitudes toward their children have all been noted to be maintained over periods of 3 months to 4.5 years and even 9 years after treatment termination (Dubey et al., 1983; Forehand & McMahon, 1981; McMahon & Forehand, 1984; Patterson, 1982; Patterson et al., 1992; Patterson & Fleischman, 1979; Pisterman et al., 1989; Strain, Steele, Ellis, & Timm, 1982; Webster-Stratton, 1982; Webster-Stratton et al., 1989). Yet, several studies have noted that parental use of positive attending skills to prosocial child behavior is less likely to be maintained at follow-up than is the parents' use of other skills taught within the program (Patterson, 1982; Webster-Stratton, 1982; Webster-Stratton et al., 1989). Despite this decline in parental positive attending skills after treatment termination, gains in child behavior found at the end of treatment continue to be maintained across follow-up periods up to 4.5 years later. This wealth of studies reflecting the maintenance of treatment gains over time is encouraging but it is not found in all research studies of parent training; a few studies have not found such long-term effects of behavioral parent training (Bernal et al., 1980; Strayhorn & Weidman, 1991), suggesting that lasting gains are not always the norm for all forms of behavioral parent training.

Generalization of Treatment Gains across Settings

Therapists, as well as school staff, may be tempted to believe that parental participation in behavioral parent training programs at the offices of mental health professionals or even in the parents' homes will result in improved child behavior at school. Unfortunately, most studies have not found such generalization of treatment gains to school settings to occur (Horn, Ialongo, Greenberg, Packard, & Smith-Winberry, 1990; Horn, Ialongo, Popovich, & Peradotto, 1987; McMahon & Forehand, 1984; Patterson, 1982), although at least one has done so (Strayhorn & Weidman, 1991). Some studies have found children whose parents received parent training, or at least a subset of such children, to manifest improved school conduct, but just as many children within those studies either showed no change in school behavior or a significant worsening of such behavior associated with parent training (Firestone, Kelly, Goodman, & Davey, 1981; McMahon & Forehand, 1984). None of the studies that failed to find generalization of treatment effects to school settings, however, directly targeted school behavior problems as part of the parent training program. Consequently, therapists using traditional behavioral parent training programs should not encourage either parents or school staff to believe that generalization of gains to child school behavior is likely to occur. This is one of the reasons why, in this edition, I have added a session to help parents assist teachers with improving their children's school conduct and performance through the use of home-based reward programs. Such procedures have been shown to result in improved teacher ratings of school behavior and improved homework performance (Atkeson & Forehand, 1978).

Predictors of Success and Failure

Research with this program suggests that up to 64% or more of families with ADHD and/or clinically serious oppositional children may expect to demonstrate clinically significant change or recovery (normalization) with this program (Anastopoulos et al., 1993; Pisterman et al., 1989; Quici, Wheeler, & Bolle, 1996) and similar such programs (Bernal et al., 1980; Dishion & Patterson, 1992; Webster-Stratton et al., 1989). The percentage improved is greater among younger (< 6 years) and less clinically severe children (Dishion & Patterson, 1992; Webster-Stratton, 1982). But not all families can be expected to benefit from a behavioral parent training program such as this one. Research on similar such programs suggests a number of factors that are related to program ineffectiveness (number of sessions attended, failure to complete training or to return for follow-up, reduced level of improvement in parent and child conflicts). Such factors should be considered by parent trainers as a possible basis on which to triage families into those assigned to group parent training (good likelihood of responding) versus individual training (higher number of risk factors), or even to divide families into those who are to be offered parent training and those who may need other, more parent-focused treatments first (Holden, Lavigne, & Cameron, 1990).

Child Factors

Only a few child characteristics have been identified as related to the effectiveness of parent training programs. As noted above, one relatively consistent predictor of diminished effectiveness of parent training is the age of the child. Preschool children (< 6 years) appear to have the highest rates (≥ 65%) of positive responding to behavioral parent training programs, compared with school-age children, who are somewhat less likely to improve (50–64%) (Anastopoulos et al., 1993; Dishion & Patterson, 1992; Strain et al., 1982; Strain, Young, & Horowitz, 1981), or with adolescents (25–35%) (Barkley, Guevremont, et al., 1992). However, this effect of age actually might be an inverted U-shaped or curvilinear function, in that within the preschool age group, higher parental drop-out rates and lesser degrees of responding have been found to be associated with *younger* ages of the children (Holden et al., 1990). And even within the elementary age range, the effect of age on treatment response has been found in one study to be the opposite of that noted above, with parents of younger children being more likely to discontinue treatment prematurely (Firestone & Witt, 1982). Higher intelligence or mental age in children has also been associated positively with better response to parent training or with parental persistence through a parent training program (Firestone & Witt, 1982).

The severity of the children's behavioral problems and defiance, specifically, has been noted in some studies as being correlated with more limited treatment efficacy and a greater likelihood of parental premature termination from training (Dumas, 1984; Holden et al., 1990). But this relationship might be explained by another one, that being the relationship of parental stress, marital distress, and parental psychopathology to the severity of the child's problems (Webster-Stratton & Hammond, 1990). That is, the severity of the child's problems here is simply serving as a marker for more important parent factors (see below) that are the actual reason parents terminate training prematurely or fail to respond positively to the training.

As noted above, children with ADHD who are also defiant and whose parents undergo this training program should not be expected to be "recovered" or normalized in all of their behavioral problems as a consequence of this program. Research suggests that child defiant and hostile behavior is likely to improve the most from this program, with ADHD symptoms improving only somewhat or not at all (Anastopoulos et al., 1993; Johnston, 1992). And so stimulant medication or other pharmacological therapy may need to be added to the treatment package provided to such children in order to address more fully the defiant child's comorbid ADHD (Firestone et al., 1981). Where stimulant medication is used with ADHD children, therapists may find that there is sometimes little additional benefit provided to families by including a parent training program (Abikoff & Hechtman, 1995; Firestone et al., 1981; Horn et al., 1991). Given that stimulant medications have proven to be among the most effective treatments for these children (Barkley, 1990; Rapport & Kelly, 1993; Swanson, McBurnett, Christian, & Wigal, 1995), clinicians should discuss this treatment with parents upon making the diagnosis of ADHD. Some parents wish to wait until after training is done, however. Thus, in this edition I have amended the original parent training program to suggest discussing this issue in the final session of the program for those parents who have elected to wait to begin such treatment. Therapists wishing more information about psychopharmacology for ADHD children are referred to texts by Werry and Aman (1993, in press), Weiss (1992), Greenhill and Osmon (1991), and myself (1990), as well as the Spring 1990 (Vol. 1, No. 1) issue of the *Journal of Child and Adolescent Psychopharmacology*.

Parent Factors

Parents who are relatively younger than the average of those seeking training, who are less intelligent and/or have less than a high school education, and who are of lower social class usually do not achieve the same degree of success as others (Dumas, 1984; Firestone & Witt, 1982; Holden et al., 1990; Knapp & Deluty, 1989; Webster-Stratton & Hammond, 1990). However, the detrimental effects of lower socioeconomic status have not always been noted in studies of behavioral parent training (McMahon & Forehand, 1984; Rogers, Forehand, Griest, Wells, & McMahon, 1981). One study also found that the family's ethnic group was associated with dropping out of treatment or progressing more slowly through training, with minority groups having more of these difficulties than the majority group (Holden et al., 1990). However, social class was also found to show the same relationship to poor progress through treatment and it, rather than ethnic group, may actually have created this difference among ethnic groups, given the differential representation of such groups across social class. As might be expected, the number of required sessions the parents actually attended in the training program has been shown to be related to treatment efficacy (Strain et al., 1981).

Diminished benefits from parent training and high drop-out rates are especially likely for parents (mothers) who are socially isolated from adult peers in their community and encounter aversive interactions with their extended family (Dumas, 1984; Dumas & Wahler, 1983; Salzinger, Kaplan, & Artemyeff, 1983; Wahler, 1980; Wahler & Afton, 1980). Even when such parents demonstrate improved child management and fewer parent–child conflicts, they may have a greater likelihood of relapse after training concludes (Dumas & Wahler, 1983; Wahler, 1980; Wahler & Afton, 1980). Dumas and Wahler (1983) have shown that maternal insularity (isolation) when combined with socioeconomic disadvantage accounted for nearly 50% of the variance in treatment effectiveness, suggesting that these factors may be particularly important during the pretreatment stage when the therapist is assessing the likelihood that a family may respond positively to behavioral parent training. It is possible, however, that by providing greater involvement and training from the therapist, ensuring more time for practice (Knapp & Deluty, 1989), and addressing the mothers' social isolation either before or during training (Dadds & McHugh, 1992; Dumas & Wahler, 1983; Wahler, Cartor, Fleischman, & Lambert, 1993), these families may be able achieve significant improvements in child management.

Parents with serious forms of psychopathology (psychosis, severe depression, alcohol/drug dependency, etc.) do not seem to do well in parent training programs such as this one (Patterson & Chamberlain, 1992). They start out resistant to training and homework assignments and seem to remain so throughout treatment. Also, parents demonstrating greater negativity and helplessness or poor anger control typically do not respond as positively in such training programs or are more likely to drop out of treatment (Frankel & Simmons, 1992). Perhaps providing training in more effective problem-solving (Pfiffner, Jouriles, Brown, Etscheidt, & Kelly, 1988; Prinz & Miller, 1994; Spaccarelli et al., 1992) or anger management skills prior to or as an adjunct to parent training in child management may prove useful in enhancing the effectiveness of parent training programs (see Goldstein, Keller, & Erne, 1985; Sanders, 1996, for a discussion).

In the coming decade, research on parent training is likely to focus increased attention on the relationship of parental ADHD to child ODD and to parental responsiveness to parent training. ADHD in children is known to have a strong hereditary predisposition (see Barkley, 1996, for discussion), with an average of 25% of immediate family members likely to have the disorder. This means that there is at least a 50% chance that *one* of the ADHD child's biological parents is an adult with ADHD. Up to 65% of children with ADHD may have ODD as a comorbid disorder, and even those who do not are likely to be more difficult to manage than are normal children, making childhood ADHD a common factor among children whose families are being recommended for a behavioral parent training program such as this one. This suggests that not only is there a significant probability that the child who is the focus of the parent training efforts has ADHD, but that one of the child's parents may have ADHD as well. Evans, Vallano, and Pelham (1994) have discussed the detrimental effects parental ADHD may have on the parent training process and have even shown that treatment of parental ADHD with stimulant medication may prove useful in facilitating a positive response of that parent to the parent training course. For these reasons, assessment instruments have been added in this edition to assist clinicians in screening for the presence of both childhood ADHD and parental ADHD in families.

Degree of marital discord is also a predictor of diminished effectiveness within this (Forehand & McMahon, 1981) and other (Patterson, 1982; Webster-Stratton & Hammond, 1990) parent training programs. Perhaps it is better to provide such parents with marital therapy (Dadds, Schwartz, & Sanders, 1987) or divorce counseling to help resolve their marital problems before parent training in child management is offered or as an adjunct to it. As might be expected, whether or not the family was intact (parents married) at the time of training is also a predictor of response to parent training programs, with single-parent families responding less well than two-parent households (Strain et al., 1981, 1982; Webster-Stratton & Hammond, 1990). Degree of life stress experienced within the past year may also be associated with reduced parent training efficacy (Webster-Stratton & Hammond, 1990).

Therapist Factors

Lately, increasing attention has been paid to the role that therapist factors may play in the success of behavioral parent training programs. Such factors long have been known to be of importance in studies of psychotherapy outcomes with adults (Garfield & Bergen, 1986) and, more recently, in psychotherapy studies with children (Crits-Christoph & Mintz, 1991; Kazdin, 1991). A few studies have examined this issue relative to behavioral parent training, particularly among Patterson's research team at the Oregon Social Learning Center. Trainee-therapists do not appear to be as effective in maintaining parents in parent training programs as are more experienced therapists (Frankel & Simmons, 1992). Moreover, among experienced therapists, those who teach and confront parents more are likely to encounter greater parent resistance to training than are those who facilitate and support parents in the process of training (Patterson & Forgatch, 1985). Resistance can occur both in response to the formal training procedures within the session as well as to the homework assignments parents are required to perform (Patterson & Chamberlain, 1992). Patterson and Chamberlain (1992) report that parent trainers working with families of seriously antisocial children can expect to encounter resistance from most families at the start of treatment, which is likely to increase up to the midpoint of treatment. In less serious cases and in families with younger children, this resistance may be worked through and resolved by the time of treatment termination. In more difficult cases, resistance is likely to persist at high levels, foreboding fewer changes in parent's management skills with their children as well as less positive outcomes overall. Such client resistance is likely to provoke the therapist into confronting behaviors, which, as noted above, may increase client resistance. Thus, a "delicate balancing act" must be achieved by the parent training therapist, who is attempting to achieve an optimal level of teaching and confronting of parents' resistance while providing facilitation and support to motivate the parents to undertake behavioral change (Patterson & Chamberlain, 1992).

Organization of the Manual

This training manual has been organized into four parts: Part I provides information on the background of this program, its theoretical and research basis, methods of evaluating oppositional and defiant children both before and after treatment, and various prerequisite information to consider before undertaking this program of therapy. Part II provides detailed instructions on conducting each of the sessions of the program. Clinicians may wish not only to acquaint themselves thoroughly with Part II but also to review the contents of each step periodically while training families. Each step in this section begins with an outline of the material to be taught in that step, such that a clinician experienced in this program need only refer to this outline during a training session with a family. Part III contains assessment materials, which are highly useful during the pre- and posttreatment evaluation of the children and their families. Part IV contains the handouts to be used with each step of the program. (Note that Parts III and IV are included in a Spanish-language supplement available from the publisher; see point 8, below.)

Revisions to the Original Program

Readers already familiar with the original manual for this program (Barkley, 1987) may appreciate knowing about the modifications presented in the second edition. Most of these changes are listed below:

1. The introductory section (above) of the manual as well as Chapter 1 ("The Rationale for the Program") are much more densely referenced with citations of the research literature that support the efficacy of the program and its components. This was done so that therapists wishing to venture into the empirical literature behind the program and its methods could do so more easily. It was also done to buttress many of the assertions set forth in the original manual for which citations had not been provided. Finally, clinicians negotiating with managed care or other insurance companies for approval of these services and remuneration of clinical fees for the training program may need to cite the clinical research literature on the proven effectiveness of behavioral parent training in support of their case for reimbursement from these companies. Photocopying appropriate sections of this manual (see the copyright page for limitations) and providing them to such managed care companies in support of such negotiations can be helpful.

2. The assessment materials have been greatly revised and expanded to include demographic information, developmental/medical history, and more thorough pa-

rental interview forms that should prove highly useful in conducting evaluations of defiant children. In particular, the parental interview is updated to include a review of all of those childhood disorders and their symptoms that are most likely to be seen in association with defiant behavior, ODD, or CD in children. In this interview, the symptoms and diagnostic criteria for these disorders are based on those described in the fourth edition of the *Diagnostic and Statistical Manual of Mental Disorders* (DSM-IV; American Psychiatric Association, 1994). Use of this interview can assist with determining the clinical diagnoses for most child referrals. New child behavior rating scales have been added that directly evaluate the symptoms of the three Disruptive Behavior Disorders from DSM-IV (ADHD, ODD, and CD) according to parent report, and two of these disorders (ADHD, ODD) by teacher report. The Home and School Situations Questionnaires are, once again, provided here to assist with identifying the precise situations in which disruptive behavior is occurring, in part to aid treatment planning but also to gain an impression of the pervasiveness of the children's behavioral problems. A scale for assessing symptoms of ADHD in parents of children is also provided, along with guidelines for the scoring and interpretation of all of these scales.

3. The original Steps 3 (Increasing Compliance) and 4 (Decreasing Disruptiveness) have been combined into a single session (Step 3) in this edition, based on our clinical experience that both can be easily covered within a single training meeting with parents.

4. This permitted the addition of a new step (now Step 8) dealing with Daily School Behavior Report Cards, which parents can use to assist teachers in improving a child's behavior and academic performance in the classroom. A new parent handout and several versions of useful daily school behavior report cards are now provided in this revised manual. Obviously, this step is intended for school-age children and can be skipped in preschool-age children.

5. The training of parents in a procedure for mild, brief spanking of their children when the children escaped from a time out location without permission has been eliminated from this edition. That procedure had been an effective part of this program since the original "two-stage" program was conceived and studied by Constance Hanf, PhD, in the 1960s at the Oregon Health Sciences University, and was retained in its iterations by others (Barkley, 1981, 1987; Forehand & McMahon, 1981; Roberts, 1982). However, over the past 30 years, societal attitudes toward the use of corporal punishment with children, even mild spanking, have shifted such that these methods are viewed as increasingly less acceptable by parents (Hefer & Kelley, 1987), especially with school-age children (Socolar & Stein, 1995). A similar trend has become evident among therapists working with families of behavior problem children (Webster-Stratton et al., 1989), in that there has been a growing disdain for teaching parents such methods. In part, this may

be founded on the belief that the use of physical punishment with children who may already be aggressive serves simply to model further aggressive behavior for the child to imitate. And in part this changing attitude may have arisen from some studies showing that physical punishment by parents significantly (though modestly) correlated with level of aggression by the children, and so it seems to be (Strassberg, Dodge, Petit, & Bates, 1994). The idea that parental use of physical punishment is *causing* the children's behavior may have become well established in both parental and clinical lore, even though correlations such as these cannot prove causality. Many factors account for such relationships, making it difficult to interpret the correlation as evidence of a straightforward cause, leading from parental mild physical discipline to childhood aggression. Research findings simply are unclear about the direction of effects in this relationship, and have not shown that it applies to the *consistent* use by parents of *mild* physical discipline, such as the brief spanking method taught in the original program. Nor have those studies held constant other important parental and family factors (e.g., parental negative beliefs about discipline, parental inconsistency in using behavior consequences, antisocial personality disorder, depression, marital discord, etc.) in most analyses of these data, which might mediate this relationship between parental discipline and child aggression (Larzelere, 1996; Socolar & Stein, 1995). Even so, the decline in social acceptance of this child management method alone would justify its removal from this program, provided, of course, that a noncorporal alternative to managing escape from time out exists. Fortunately, that alternative has been developed and found to be equally as efficacious (Day & Roberts, 1982), and so it has been substituted here. That method involves the use of a barrier restraint, such as isolation of the child to his/her bedroom and closing and locking the door if necessary to preclude escape from time out.

6. The original Step 8 of this program ("Managing Noncompliance in Public Places") is now covered in Step 7 and has been broadened to include the use of "think aloud–think ahead" steps by parents in places other than just public ones. It also incorporates the use of "planned activities" as a preventive measure to ward off the likelihood of child behavior problems in immediately upcoming home and public situations.

7. The contents of some of the parent handouts have been slightly modified in accordance with the above changes, as well as to include additional helpful information and procedures. In a few cases, the wording of these handouts has been improved upon to clarify how parents should carry out the particular procedure under discussion when used at home.

8. And finally, a Spanish translation of the assessment tools and parent handouts has been created as a separate supplement to this manual that is available from the publisher.

Summary

The procedures detailed in this manual are designed specifically for families with children who are noncompliant, defiant, or oppositional and who range in age from 2 to 12 years. The methods are meant for use by experienced clinicians with adequate training in delivering psychological services to families of defiant children. Although highly effective, the success of these procedures is dependent on the nature and severity of the child's problems, the child's age, the extent and severity of parental and family psychopathology, and the level of parental intelligence and motivation to utilize these methods, among other factors. When taught properly, this program can be significantly effective in diminishing or eliminating behavior problems in children.

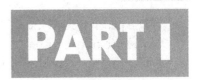

PART I

Prerequisite Information for Using the Program

CHAPTER 1

The Rationale for the Program

This chapter presents the primary focus of the parent training program, the rationale behind selecting this focus, and the important findings from research supporting this focus. As Mash and Terdal (1996) have stated, the target of behavioral assessment and treatment must be clearly defined, have relevance to the presenting complaints of the child and family, have significance for the child's present and future adjustment, and, where possible, be grounded in an adequate theory of its development and maintenance. The target of this intervention program, *child noncompliance and defiance*, clearly meets these requirements (Forehand & McMahon, 1981).

Noncompliance Defined

The term "noncompliance" as used here will refer to three categories of child behavior, these being the following:

1. The child's failure to initiate behaviors requested by an adult within a reasonable time after a command given by that adult. In most cases, a reasonable time refers to 15 seconds after the command was given, although parents may specifically stipulate when compliance is to be initiated (e.g., "As soon as that cartoon is over, pick up your toys!"). Research on noncompliance has generally used a more stringent interval of 10 seconds after a command was given as a reasonable time for compliance to be initiated.

2. The child's failure to sustain compliance to a command from an adult until the requirements stipulated in the command have been fulfilled. Some may consider this behavior category as a form of attention span or sustained attention to tasks ("on-task" behavior).

3. The child's failure to follow previously taught rules of conduct in a situation. Such behaviors as leaving one's desk in class or running off in a department store without permission, stealing, lying, hitting or aggressing against others, taking food from the kitchen without permission, and swearing at one's parents are just a few child behaviors that parents consider to be violations of previously taught standards of conduct.

The term "noncompliance," however, may convey the notion of passive avoidance of completing parental commands and requests or following previously stated household rules. Thus, the term "defiance" can also be used for many instances of noncompliant behavior where the child displays active verbal or physical resistance to complying with such parental directives, as in the case of verbal refusal, temper outbursts, and even physically aggressing against a parent when the parent attempts to impose compliance with a directive on the child. Examples of noncompliant and defiant behaviors are shown in Table 1.1. Despite their apparent dissimilarity, all of these behaviors can be construed as belonging to a more general or larger class of behavior that involves noncompliance, or what some have called hostile–defiant behavior or social aggression. Some of the behaviors in Table 1.1 are in fact direct efforts of the child to escape or avoid the imposition of the command (see Patterson, 1982). Hence, all may be treated by a common program that addresses noncompliance. Research has shown that treating noncompliance often results in significant improvements in other behaviors in this general class even though those behaviors were not specifically targeted by the intervention (Russo, Cataldo, & Cushing, 1981; Wells, Forehand, & Griest, 1980). It is this targeting of noncompliance that distinguishes this parent training program from many others, which may single out one or several types of inappropriate behavior but fail to address the more general class of noncompliance to which such specific forms of noncompliance belong.

Another means of understanding the relationships among various forms of disruptive behavior comes from meta-analytic reviews of the literature that have employed factor analysis to study these relationships. One such review by Frick et al. (1993) resulted in a figure, reprinted here in Figure 1.1, that shows how various forms of oppositional behavior may

TABLE 1.1. Types of Noncompliant Behaviors Common in Children Referred for Behavior Disorders

Yells	Steals	Fails to complete routine chores
Whines	Lies	Destroys property
Complains	Argues	Physically fights with others
Defies	Humiliates/annoys	Fails to complete school homework
Screams	Teases	Disrupts others' activities
Tantrums	Ignores requests	Ignores self-care tasks
Throws objects	Runs off	
Talks back	Cries	
Swears	Physically resists	

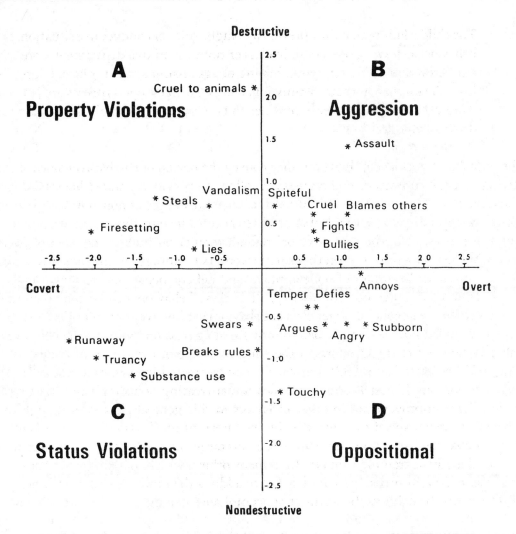

FIGURE 1.1. A diagram representing the results of a meta-analysis of factor analytic studies of disruptive child behavior. From Frick et al. (1993, p. 327). Copyright 1993 by Pergamon Press. Reprinted by permission.

cluster into a form of overt disruptive behavior that is nondestructive but is related to three other equally, if not more serious, forms of antisocial acts, status violations, and aggression toward and offenses against others. The diagram suggests that we can classify defiant children into four somewhat separable groups based on this two-dimensional system (Overt–Covert, Nondestructive–Destructive). Although not obvious from the diagram, there is a developmental staging or relationship among these subgroups, discussed later. This supports the point to be made later in this chapter that childhood oppositional behavior carries significant developmental risks for the progression of the child into more serious forms of conduct disorder, as well as antisocial and even criminal activity (Lahey & Loeber, 1994; Lahey, Loeber, Quay, Frick, & Grimm, 1992; Loeber, 1988, 1990).

When Is Treatment Justified?

Some noncompliant or defiant behavior is normal for children, particularly those in the preschool age group, and should not be thought of as being pathological or abnormal just because it may occur sporadically. Nor will such typical and occasional defiance justify a clinical treatment program such as this one. Clinicians must take care to establish *at least two of the following three criteria* for determining that the noncompliant behavior shown by a child referred to them can be justified as in need of clinical intervention:

1. The child's behavior is developmentally inappropriate or statistically deviant in that it occurs to a significantly greater degree than is common for children of this age group. This can be established through the use of child behavior rating scales that include this dimension of behavior, often called aggression or conduct problem by scale developers. More will be said about such assessment methods in Chapter 2. For now, suffice it to say that the child's behavior should be rated as falling at least above the 84th percentile (1 standard deviation [*SD*] above the mean) or higher on such rating scales in order to establish such deviance. Although this information will typically be obtained through the use of parent reports of the child's behavior because the home setting is where such behavior is usually at its worst, teacher reports on these rating scales may also be used to establish this criterion of developmental inappropriateness. Alternatively, through clinical interview with the parent one can discover whether the child demonstrates sufficient symptoms of ODD or CD as to meet clinical criteria for either of these diagnoses as established in DSM-IV (American Psychiatric Association, 1994).

2. The child's behavior is resulting in an appreciable degree of impairment. That is, the behavior pattern is interfering with the child's capacity to meet appropriate developmental expectations for adaptive behavior, such as self-care, appropriate social interaction with family members and peers, acceptance of age-appropriate responsibilities as in chore and homework performance, and the capacity to be trusted to adhere to rules in the absence of immediate caregiver (typically parental) supervision. Such levels of impairment can also be established through some child behavior rating scales that measure dimensions of adaptive behavior or through interviews and inventories that explicitly assess adaptive functioning, such as the Vineland Adaptive Behavior Scale, the Normative Adaptive Behavior Scale, or other such instruments, to be discussed further in Chapter 2. What the clinician is attempting to demonstrate is that a significant discrepancy exists between this child's general cognitive ability or intelligence and his/her adaptive functioning as measured by these instruments, so as to demonstrate that a social/adaptive disability or impairment exists in this child. A similar approach has been discussed by others for establishing the existence of a social disability in children with ADHD (Greene et al., 1996; Roizen, Blondis, Irwin, & Stein, 1994). For our purposes, establishing that a defiant child's adaptive functioning places him/her at or below the 10th percentile for his/her age would be reasonably sufficient for this purpose.

This approach is similar to establishing an IQ–academic achievement score discrepancy as a partial basis for defining the presence of a learning disability.

3. The child's behavior is resulting in a significant degree of emotional distress or harm, either for the child or, more likely, for the parents, siblings, or peers of this child. Child distress may be established through the use of child self-report measures of emotional adjustment, such as ratings of anxiety or depression, that convey an impression of the child's unhappiness with the current state of affairs in the family specifically or their social adjustment more generally. Parent distress may be readily established most directly through the use of parent self-report instruments designed to measure this domain, such as the Short Form of the Parenting Stress Index (Abidin, 1986). Distress to peers can be established through rating scales of social skills and peer acceptance completed by parents or teachers.

Regardless of the specific methods used to evaluate these intervention criteria, the clinician must make some effort to demonstrate that the child's defiant behavior pattern is outside the bounds of normally appropriate child conduct and that it is impairing the child's adjustment in some way or is creating distress for the child, the caregiver, or others and thus is in need of clinical intervention. Statistical deviance of a child's behavior alone may not justify either clinical diagnosis or clinical intervention. It may be helpful here to consider the related issue of what defines a behavior pattern as a mental disorder, out of which may come some guidance concerning the issue of when to treat. As discussed by Wakefield (1992), the clinician is attempting to establish that a "harmful dysfunction" exists and is deserving of a label of mental disorder and/or clinical treatment. Wakefield (1992) goes further and requires that an aberration in an internal, normal mental or cognitive mechanism must also be present to define a "harmful dysfunction"; this must be shown before a diagnosis of mental disorder is rendered. As Richters and Cichetti (1993) have argued, some defiant or antisocial children may show no evidence of aberrant cognitive mechanisms, although many do (see Hinshaw & Anderson, 1996, for a review), and their deviant behavior may arise as a result of external mechanisms, such as criminogenic environments. Such children may not be viewed as having mental disorders. Others disagree with Wakefield's criterion of an aberrant cognitive mechanism (Lilienfeld & Marino, 1995), however, and argue that "fuzzy" boundaries will invariably exist between normality and abnormality by virtue of the dimensional nature of individual psychological characteristics and behaviors and because one must make arbitrary choices about "where to carve nature at her joints" to define abnormality along any dimension (see also Mash & Dozois, 1996). Also, I am not sure that a criterion of an aberrant internal mechanism or even a diagnosis of mental disorder is needed to justify the use of psychosocial treatment for the child and his/her parent. Some relatively socially benign interventions, such as parent training in child management, may be justifiable even though some children whose parents undergo such training do not meet diagnostic thresholds for a mental disorder or Wakefield's complete criteria for a "harmful dysfunction." The implementation of treatment, in other words, may not necessarily depend on a diagnosis of a mental disorder, although often it does.

In the end, what all of this means is that the clinician must stay alert to the occasional possibility that some children and their families do not need specific child management training. This may result from the fact that some parents, by dint of their own psychological or psychiatric disorders, are significantly distressed by even normal, garden-variety child misbehavior or noncompliance. In such cases, parents may need intervention for changing their own distress (and developmental expectations of children) rather than the child's behavior needing clinical treatment. Milder instances of this phenomenon, where parents manifest no serious psychological disorders, may simply reflect an excess of parental concern about their children's adjustment and their own competence as parents. In these cases, the clinician may only need to offer simple reassurance that all seems well with the child and that the parent seems to be doing a reasonable job of parenting. Likewise, some children may show higher than normal levels of oppositional behavior that do not achieve clinically significant levels of deviance, result in no distress for the parent or child, or are not associated with significant impairment in adaptive functioning. Such children may be viewed as more stubborn, "pig-headed," strong-willed, temperamental, rigid, or opinionated but such personality descriptors alone would not justify clinical intervention. And there certainly exist those rare cases of children who may be distressed by their own social conduct, even though not clinically deviant in their noncompliance, not distressing to their parents, or/and not impaired in their adaptive functioning, as in the case of Social Phobia, Major Depressive Disorder, Dysthymic Disorder, or even Obsessive–Compulsive Disorder. Such children may well be in need of clinical treatment for their own psychological distress but not specifically in need of a parent training program aimed at noncompliant child behavior management as that described here. But the presence of at least two of the three criteria set forth above is likely to indicate that a child's behavior is placing him/her at significant risk for current and later maladjustment, social and academic failure, antisocial activities, and other significant negative developmental outcomes. This establishes that a "harmful dysfunction" exists (even if not associated with an aberrant cognitive mechanism) and that such adaptational risks justify clinical intervention.

Degrees of Noncompliance/Defiance

As the foregoing discussion makes apparent, there exist degrees of noncompliant behavior, the terms for which do not always have a consensus of professional opinion. Whereas degrees of intellectual deficits may be carved into categories of slow, borderline, mild, moderate, and severe or profound to define mental retardation, no such consensus exists for labeling degrees of noncompliant or defiant behavior, though adapting some of the former categories might be appropriate for a dimension of defiant behavior. On a well-standardized behavior rating scale of this dimension, children whose defiant behavior exceeds the mean by only one standard deviation ($+1\,SD$, 84th percentile) or less are considered normal even though possibly being stubborn or strong-willed. Those children placing above the 84th percentile but below the 93rd percentile (within $+1$ to $+1.5\,SD$) could be described as being "noncompliant" (Forehand & McMahon, 1981) or "difficult," or as having borderline ODD, provided they do not meet the full clinical diagnostic criteria for that

TABLE 1.2. Diagnostic Criteria for Oppositional Defiant Disorder

A. A pattern of negativistic, hostile, and defiant behavior lasting at least 6 months, during which four (or more) of the following are present:

   (1) often loses temper
   (2) often argues with adults
   (3) often actively defies or refuses to comply with adults' requests or rules
   (4) often deliberately annoys people
   (5) often blames others for his or her mistakes or misbehavior
   (6) is often touchy or easily annoyed by others
   (7) is often angry and resentful
   (8) is often spiteful or vindictive

Note: Consider a criterion met only if the behavior occurs more frequently than is typically observed in individuals of comparable age and developmental level.

B. The disturbance in behavior causes clinically significant impairment in social, academic, or occupational functioning.

C. The behaviors do not occur exclusively during the course of a Psychotic or Mood Disorder.

D. Criteria are not met for Conduct Disorder, and, if the individual is age 18 years or older, criteria are not met for Antisocial Personality Disorder.

Note. From American Psychiatric Association (1994, pp. 93–94). Copyright 1994 by the American Psychiatric Association. Reprinted by permission.

disorder in the DSM-IV. Those children who place above the 93rd percentile on such rating scales or who meet full clinical criteria for ODD by the DSM-IV diagnostic rules would be said to have that disorder, perhaps further qualified as mild, moderate, or severe depending on the severity of their ratings of deviant behavior on the rating scales or the number of ODD symptoms they possess above the minimal number required to meet the diagnostic threshold. Children in most of these categories except the normal one might be appropriate for this parent training program, provided that the criteria for justifying intervention described above were met.

For those unfamiliar with the current clinical diagnostic criteria for ODD and its more severe counterpart, CD, as set forth in DSM-IV (American Psychiatric Association, 1994), these are provided in Tables 1.2 and 1.3. Considering that the majority of children with ODD and CD often have ADHD as a comorbid condition, the diagnostic criteria for that disorder are provided as well, in Table 1.4. Clinicians wishing to become more familiar with that disorder and its treatment will find the texts by myself (1990, 1996), Hinshaw (1994), Matson (1993), Weiss (1992), and Weiss and Hechtman (1993) to be quite informative.

As noted earlier, childhood ODD is strongly associated with risk for eventual childhood CD (Lahey & Loeber, 1994; Lahey et al., 1992; Patterson, 1982; Patterson et al., 1992). Although approximately 20–25% of children with ODD may no longer have the disorder 3 years later, up to 52% will persist in having ODD over this period of time. Of those who persist with ODD, nearly half (25% of the initial total of ODD children) will progress into childhood CD within a 3-year follow-up period (Lahey et al., 1992). However, among

TABLE 1.3. Diagnostic Criteria for Conduct Disorder

A. A repetitive and persistent pattern of behavior in which the basic rights of others or major age-appropriate societal norms or rules are violated, as manifested by the presence of three (or more) of the following criteria in the past 12 months, with at least one criterion present in the past 6 months:

Aggression to people and animals
(1) often bullies, threatens, or intimidates others
(2) often initiates physical fights
(3) has used a weapon that can cause serious physical harm to others (e.g., a bat, brick, broken bottle, knife, gun)
(4) has been physically cruel to people
(5) has been physically cruel to animals
(6) has stolen while confronting a victim (e.g., mugging, purse snatching, extortion, armed robbery)
(7) has forced someone into sexual activity

Destruction of property
(8) has deliberately engaged in fire setting with the intention of causing serious damage
(9) has deliberately destroyed others' property (other than by fire setting)

Deceitfulness or theft
(10) has broken into someone else's house, building, or car
(11) often lies to obtain goods or favors or to avoid obligations (i.e., "cons" others)
(12) has stolen items of nontrivial value without confronting a victim (e.g., shoplifting, but without breaking and entering; forgery)

Serious violations of rules
(13) often stays out at night despite parental prohibitions, beginning before age 13 years
(14) has run away from home overnight at least twice while living in parental or parental surrogate home (or once without returning for a lengthy period)
(15) is often truant from school, beginning before age 13 years

B. The disturbance in behavior causes clinically significant impairment in social, academic, or occupational functioning.

C. If the individual is age 18 years or older, criteria are not met for Antisocial Personality Disorder.

Specify type based on age at onset:
  Childhood-Onset Type: onset of at least one criterion characteristic of Conduct Disorder prior to age 10 years
  Adolescent-Onset Type: absence of any criteria characteristic of Conduct Disorder prior to age 10 years

Specify severity:
  Mild: few if any conduct problems in excess of those required to make the diagnosis and conduct problems cause only minor harm to others
  Moderate: number of conduct problems and effect on others intermediate between "mild" and "severe"
  Severe: many conduct problems in excess of those required to make the diagnosis **or** conduct problems cause considerable harm to others

Note. From American Psychiatric Association (1994, pp. 90–91). Copyright 1994 by the American Psychiatric Association. Reprinted by permission.

children who progress into CD, over 80% will have had ODD as a preexisting disorder (Lahey et al., 1992), making ODD the most common early developmental stage for the later progression into CD. And so, while the majority of ODD children will not progress further into CD, children with persistent ODD are more likely to do so, and the vast majority of children with CD will have come to this end by way of earlier ODD. Others have documented similar developmental pathways into CD, although variations on these pathways exist and are related to the type of CD likely to emerge later in development (Lahey & Loeber, 1994; Loeber, 1988, 1990; Loeber et al., 1993; Patterson et al., 1992).

TABLE 1.4. Diagnostic Criteria for Attention-Deficit/Hyperactivity Disorder

A. Either (1) or (2):

   (1) six (or more) of the following symptoms of **inattention** have persisted for at least 6 months to a degree that is maladaptive and inconsistent with developmental level:

   Inattention
   (a) often fails to give close attention to details or makes careless mistakes in schoolwork, work, or other activities
   (b) often has difficulty sustaining attention in tasks or play activities
   (c) often does not seem to listen when spoken to directly
   (d) often does not follow through on instructions and fails to finish schoolwork, chores, or duties in the workplace (not due to oppositional behavior or failure to understand instructions)
   (e) often has difficulty organizing tasks and activities
   (f) often avoids, dislikes, or is reluctant to engage in tasks that require sustained mental effort (such as schoolwork or homework)
   (g) often loses things necessary for tasks or activities (e.g., toys, school assignments, pencils, books, or tools)
   (h) is often easily distracted by extraneous stimuli
   (I) is often forgetful in daily activities

   (2) six (or more) of the following symptoms of **hyperactivity–impulsivity** have persisted for at least 6 months to a degree that is maladaptive and inconsistent with developmental level:

   Hyperactivity
   (a) often fidgets with hands or feet or squirms in seat
   (b) often leaves seat in classroom or in other situations in which remaining seated is expected
   (c) often runs about or climbs excessively in situations in which it is inappropriate (in adolescents or adults, may be limited to subjective feelings of restlessness)
   (d) often has difficulty playing or engaging in leisure activities quietly
   (e) is often "on the go" or often acts as if "driven by a motor"
   (f) often talks excessively

   Impulsivity
   (g) often blurts out answers before the questions have been completed
   (h) often has difficulty awaiting turn
   (I) often interrupts or intrudes on others (e.g., butts into conversations or games)

B. Some hyperactive–impulsive or inattentive symptoms that caused impairment were present before age 7 years.

C. Some impairment from the symptoms is present in two or more settings (e.g., at school [or work] and at home).

D. There must be clear evidence of clinically significant impairment in social, academic, or occupational functioning.

E. The symptoms do not occur exclusively during the course of a Pervasive Developmental Disorder, Schizophrenia, or other Psychotic Disorder, and are not better accounted for by another mental disorder (e.g., Mood Disorder, Anxiety Disorder, Dissociative Disorder, or a Personality Disorder).

Code based on type:
   314.01 Attention-Deficit/Hyperactivity Disorder, Combined Type: if both Criteria A1 and A2 are met for the past 6 months
   314.00 Attention-Deficit/Hyperactivity Disorder, Predominantly Inattentive Type: if Criterion A1 is met but Criterion A2 is not met for the past 6 months
   314.01 Attention-Deficit/Hyperactivity Disorder, Predominantly Hyperactive–Impulsive Type: if Criterion A2 is met but Criterion A1 is not met for the past 6 months.

Coding note: For individuals (especially adolescents and adults) who currently have symptoms that no longer meet full criteria, "In Partial Remission" should be specified.

Note. From American Psychiatric Association (1994, pp. 83–85). Copyright 1994 by the American Psychiatric Association. Reprinted by permission.

The age of onset of early CD symptoms has been shown repeatedly to be a particularly important predictor of the progression into delinquency and the severity and persistence of such delinquency, with onset of initial symptoms before age 12 years being a particularly salient threshold in making such predictions (Loeber, 1988, 1990; Loeber, Green, Lahey, Christ, & Frick, 1992; Patterson, 1982, Patterson et al., 1992; Tolan, 1987).

Prevalence of Noncompliant/Defiant Behavior

As the foregoing discussion implies, the frequency with which children manifest clinically significant and impairing levels of defiant and noncompliant behavior is greatly determined by the definition used for such disorders when surveying childhood populations. DSM-IV cites a prevalence ranging between 2 and 16% for ODD (American Psychiatric Association, 1994). For CD, rates of 6–16% for males and 2–9% for females have been cited (American Psychiatric Association, 1994). Using parent reports of child behavior problems in a large sample (1,096) of military dependents ages 6–17 years, one study (Jensen et al., 1995) reported a prevalence of 4.9% for ODD and 1.9% for CD based on diagnostic criteria from the DSM-III-R (American Psychiatric Association, 1987). Relying only on teacher ratings of DSM-III-R symptoms for a sample of 931 5–14-year-old boys, Pelham, Gnagy, Greenslade, and Milich (1992) reported a prevalence of 3.2% for ODD and 1.3% for CD. Given the limited contexts in which teachers observe child behavior (school grounds) and that oppositional and antisocial behavior is more likely to occur at home and in the community, such prevalence rates probably underestimate these disorders in the population. Another study using multiple sources of information (parent, child, teacher) for a large sample of 11-year-olds reported prevalence rates of 5.7% for ODD and 3.4% for CD (aggressive type) using DSM-III diagnostic criteria (Anderson, Williams, McGee, & Silva, 1987). In this age group, the male-to-female ratio for ODD was 2.2:1 while that for CD was 3.2:1. For adolescent samples, prevalence rates have ranged from 1.7 to 2.5% for ODD and 3.2 to 7.3% for CD, using parents' and adolescents' self-reports of symptoms based on DSM-III or DSM-III-R diagnostic criteria (Fergusson, Horwood, & Lynskey, 1993; Lewinsohn, Hops, Roberts, Seeley, & Andrews, 1993; McGee, Feehan, Williams, Partridge, Silva, & Kelly, 1990). Note the sharp decline in the prevalence of ODD but the increase in CD relative to the childhood prevalence rates for these disorders cited above. This likely attests to the fact that some ODD children are maturing out of their disorder while others show a progression of ODD into CD. Sex ratios in these samples were approximately 2:1 to 3:1 (males to females) for both ODD and CD. Both disorders, therefore, occur more commonly in males than in females but ratios vary widely as a function of both definitions and age (American Psychiatric Association, 1994; Hinshaw & Anderson, 1996), with one review suggesting that females may "catch up" with males in the their prevalence of CD by the adolescent years (Zoccolillo, 1993). Obviously, less clinically serious degrees of defiant behavior could be expected to occur with even greater frequency than these figures suggest.

Rationale for Treating Noncompliance/Defiance

This program does not simply focus on child noncompliance or defiance, but on those social processes in the family believed to have helped, at least partially, to develop or sustain the child's oppositional behavior. These processes are more thoroughly explained below in the section on the "Causes of Noncompliance/Defiance in Children." Noncompliance is the most obvious product of these social processes, although there are other significant correlates and outcomes of these processes, such as maternal depression, parental stress and low self-esteem, lack of a sense of parental competence, marital discord, and even sibling hostility and resentment, to name but a few (Forehand & McMahon, 1981; Patterson, 1982; Patterson et al., 1992). There are many well-established reasons for choosing noncompliance, and its underlying family processes, as the focus of intervention.

High Proportion of Clinic Referrals

First, noncompliance, or defiance, in various forms appears to be the most frequent complaint of families referring children to child mental health centers, especially for boys (Johnson, Wahl, Martin, & Johansson, 1973; Patterson, 1976, 1982; Patterson et al., 1992). Over half of all referrals to such clinics are for oppositional or aggressive behavior and this figure rises to more than 74% if symptoms of ADHD are included in the analysis (Patterson et al., 1993). Although these children may receive various diagnoses of ODD, CD, ADHD, Adjustment Reactions, and so forth, a major concern of the parents or teachers referring such a child is his/her inability to comply with directions, commands, rules, or codes of social conduct appropriate to the child's age group. Parents may complain that the child fails to listen, throws temper tantrums, is aggressive or destructive, is verbally oppositional or resistant to authority, fails to do homework, does not adequately perform chores, cannot play appropriately with neighborhood children, lies or steals frequently, or engages in other forms of inappropriate behavior. However, all of these behaviors are violations of commands, directions, or rules that were either previously stated to the child or are directly stated in the particular situation. Hence, noncompliance, broadly defined, encompasses the majority of acting-out, externalizing, or conduct problem forms of behavior.

High Levels of Family Conflict

Second, noncompliance underlies the majority of negative interactions between family members and the referred child. Patterson (1976, 1982; Patterson et al., 1992) and others (see Forehand & McMahon, 1981) have shown that disruptive or aggressive behavior from children occurs neither continuously nor randomly throughout the day but instead appears in "bursts" or "chunks." These are high-rate, often intense episodes of oppositional or coercive behaviors by the child that punctuate an otherwise normal stream of behavior. Research suggests that one of the most common precipitants of child noncompliance or

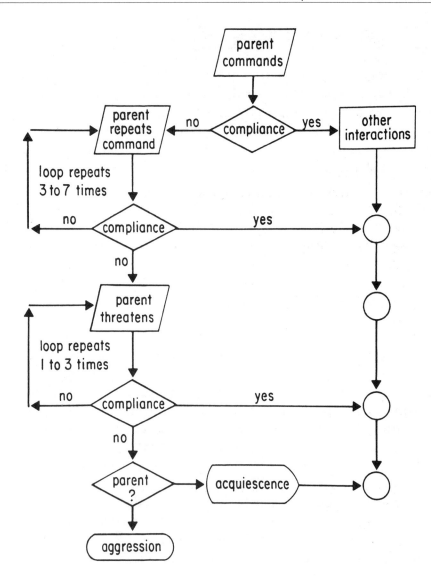

FIGURE 1.2. Flow chart showing possible sequencing of interactions between parents and defiant children during a command–compliance encounter. From Barkley (1981, p. 100). Copyright 1981 by The Guilford Press. Reprinted by permission.

defiance is parental or teacher commands or requests (Forehand & Scarboro, 1975; Green et al., 1979; Patterson, 1982; Snyder & Brown, 1983; Williams & Forehand, 1984).

Such negative encounters between adult and child seem to take the form of that shown schematically in Figure 1.2 in many, though not all, instances. The sequence is initiated by the command given by a parent, typically to have the child engage in a task that is not considered enjoyable or reinforcing by the child, such as to have the child pick up his/her toys, clean up his/her room, or perform school homework. On rare occasions, the behavior disordered child may obey this first request. This usually occurs where the command involves some very brief amount of effort or work from the child (e.g., "Please hand me a Kleenex.") or involves an activity generally pleasurable to the child or that may promise immediate reinforcement for compliance (e.g., "Get in the car so we can go get some ice cream"). In these instances, as shown by the right side of Figure 1.2, the child probably complies with the request and the family proceeds into other interactions. This may not seem especially important but what is actually significant here is the fact that rarely is such compliance followed by social reinforcement, such as a positive reaction from the parent that acknowledges appreciation for the compliance. When such compliance goes unnoted by parents, it frequently declines in occurrence over time and may eventually only occur where the activity requested of the child involves something highly intrinsically rewarding and immediately available to the child. In such cases the child obeys not because of being previously reinforced by the parent for doing so but because the specific activity required of the child is itself highly reinforcing. However, it is often only in a minority of instances that behavior disordered children will comply with the first commands or requests of parents.

More often, the pattern of events is that seen on the left side of Figure 1.2. Here the child has failed to comply with the initial command, which is often followed by the parent simply repeating the command to the child. This is rarely met with compliance from the child and so the command may be repeated again, over and over perhaps as many as 5 to 15 times (or more!) in various forms yet without the child complying with any of them. At some point, parental frustration arises and the emotional intensity of the interaction heightens. The parent may then issue a warning or threat to the child that if compliance does not occur, something unpleasant or punitive will follow. Yet, the child often fails to comply with the threat, in part, perhaps, because the parents frequently repeat it. In so doing, the threats lack credibility and often go unenforced as well. Over time, both parent and child escalate in their level of emotional behavior toward each other, with voices rising in volume and intensity, as well as collateral behavioral displays of anger, defiance, or destructiveness being shown. Ultimately, the interaction sequence ends in one of several ways. Less frequently, the parent disciplines the child, perhaps by sending the child to his/her room, removing a favored privilege from the child, or even hitting the child. Such discipline often fails because it is inconsistently applied and is delayed well past the point where compliance was initially requested. More often, the parent acquiesces and the command is left uncompleted or only partially completed by the child. Even if the task is eventually done, however, the child has succeeded in at least delaying its completion, allowing greater time for play or some other desired activity.

This latter circumstance (eventual child compliance) may prove quite an enigma to parents and therapists alike. That is, parents may believe that they have actually "won," or succeeded in getting the child to listen, yet they are surprised to find that the child will again attempt to avoid or defy that same command when issued again later. Parents may question the therapist as to why the child continues to misbehave or defy them when he ultimately will be forced to perform the task. The key to understanding this situation, however, is to see it from a child's point of view rather than an adult's. Adults tend to look at this situation in its entirety and are able to see that ultimately they will always make the child perform this command (e.g., "Get ready for bed"). Most children, however, will not show this breadth of awareness of the entire interaction sequence, but instead will simply view it as a moment-to-moment interaction with their parents in which their immediate goal is to escape or avoid doing the requested task, even if only for the moment. As a result, every minute the child is able to procrastinate is an additional minute they may continue to do what they were doing prior to the imposition of the command—an activity often more reinforcing to the child than what the parents may wish him/her to do. It is also an additional minute of avoiding the often unpleasant task requested by the parent; avoidance of unpleasant or aversive activities is itself a (negative) reinforcer for behavior.

This may help to explain why parents are often puzzled that the child spends more time avoiding the requested task, as well as arguing or defying the parents, than it would have taken to do it. The moment-by-moment procrastination of the child is doubly reinforcing in this sense, serving to permit continued participation in a desired activity (positive reinforcement) while, for the moment, successfully avoiding the unpleasant task being imposed by the parent (negative reinforcement). The ultimate outcome of the interaction (eventual punishment or forced compliance) is sufficiently delayed so as to have little, if any, influence on the child's immediate behavior.

Acquiescence occurs when the child fails to accomplish the requested activity. In some instances, the child leaves the situation. He/she may run out of the room or yard without accomplishing the task. Or the parent may storm out of the room in anger or frustration, leaving the child to return to his/her previous activities. In some cases, a parent may in fact complete the command him/herself, as is seen when a parent picks up the toys for the child. Or the parent may assist the child with the task after directing the child to do it alone. In a few instances, the child may not only succeed in escaping from doing the task, but also receive some positive consequence as well. This can be seen in cases where, for example, a mother directs a child to pick up toys, the child refuses, throws him/herself to the floor, and begins hitting his/her head against the floor. The mother may respond to this behavioral display out of fear that the child may injure him/herself, by picking the child up and holding him/her in her lap while trying to soothe the child's feelings. As a result, the child's tantrum and self-injurious behavior are not only negatively reinforced by escaping from the unpleasant task initially requested by the mother, but also are positively reinforced by the soothing attention. It is likely that such dual consequences for oppositional behavior rapidly accelerate children's acquisition and maintenance of such behavior patterns in future similar circumstances (Patterson, 1976, 1982). These acquiescent interaction patterns can be found to underlie many of the negative encounters between parents and defiant or noncompliant children. They must be the focus of treatment if the complaints of the family are to be successfully ameliorated.

Situational Pervasiveness

A third rationale for selecting noncompliance as the target of intervention is its relatively greater pervasiveness across settings compared to other behavioral problems seen in children. Research (Forehand & McMahon, 1981; Hinshaw & Anderson, 1996; Patterson, 1982) suggests that children who display noncompliance or coercive behavior in one situation are highly likely to employ it eventually elsewhere, with other commands or instructions, and with other adults or children. Improving child compliance may therefore have more widespread effects across many situations and individuals than would be seen had a behavioral problem specific to only one situation been selected as the focus of therapy.

Effects on Family Social Ecology

Fourth, noncompliant behavior by the child as outlined in Figure 1.2 may have indirect effects on family functioning that may, in a reciprocal fashion, come back to have further detrimental effects on the psychological adjustment of the defiant child. The outcomes of impaired family management as illustrated in Figure 1.2 can be seen in Figure 1.3, as demonstrated in the long-term program of research on aggressive children by Gerald Patterson (1982). As noted already, out of this impaired family management process, the child rapidly acquires a set of coercive behaviors to use against the parent and other family members or even peers when the child is instructed to do something he/she does not like to do (Patterson, 1982). Parents may also come to acquire a set of rapidly escalating coercive behaviors to use with the child because of those rare occasions where yelling, threatening, or punishing the child has eventually led to compliance by the child. Furthermore, over time parents may come to request progressively fewer commands of the child, knowing in advance they will be met with resistant, oppositional behavior by the child. Parents instead may assume more of the child's chores and responsibilities or assign them to a more compliant sibling. The latter situation may then lead not only to declines in the child's overall level of successful adaptive functioning (i.e., independence, self-care, degree of responsibleness, etc.) but to siblings developing hostility and resentment toward the defiant child because that child has comparatively less work to do. In other cases, parents and siblings come to spend progressively less leisure time and initiate fewer recreational pursuits with the defiant child so as to avoid any further unpleasantries with that child. Siblings may also acquire and frequently utilize repertoires of coercive behavior back toward the defiant child as well as toward parents (Patterson, 1982; Snyder & Patterson, 1995; Stormont-Spurgin & Zentall, 1995), given that parents may frequently employ similar coercive tactics with other members of the family and not just the clinic-referred defiant child. Thus, the density of aversive social events within the families of defiant children is substantially higher than normal. That such family patterns might have negative effects on one's self-esteem as a parent, on family harmony, on marital harmony should the child oppose one parent more than the other, or on the self-esteem of the defiant child almost goes without saying and has been substantiated in research (Forehand & McMahon, 1981; Patterson, 1982; Patterson et al., 1992). And so there is a reciprocal system of effects existing within parent–child relations of defiant children where

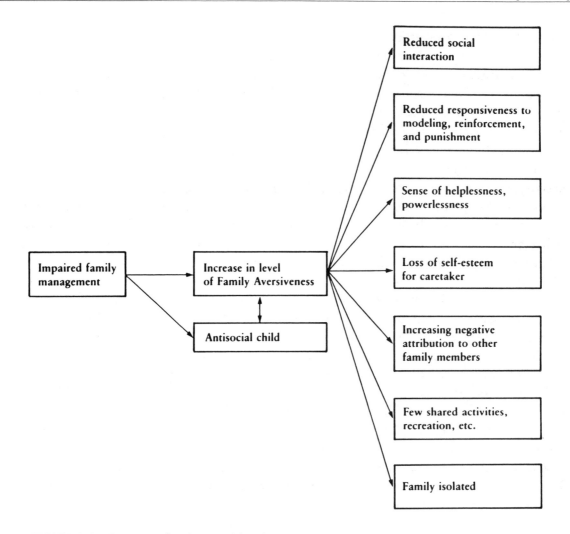

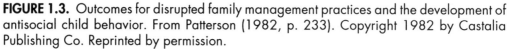

FIGURE 1.3. Outcomes for disrupted family management practices and the development of antisocial child behavior. From Patterson (1982, p. 233). Copyright 1982 by Castalia Publishing Co. Reprinted by permission.

the behavior of parent and child affect each other bidirectionally while also resulting in broader "spillover" into the larger social ecology of the family (Patterson et al., 1992; Stormont-Spurgin & Zentall, 1995; Vuchinich, Bank, & Patterson, 1992).

Developmental Persistence

Fifth, noncompliance and defiant behavior in children appears to be highly stable over time, significantly predicting the persistence of this behavior pattern across development (Fischer, Barkley, Fletcher, & Smallish, 1993; Loeber, 1990; Olweus, 1979; Patterson, 1982). Childhood defiance or aggressiveness, in fact, may be one of the most stable of childhood behavioral disorders across development.

Prediction of Diverse Negative Developmental Outcomes

Targeting early defiant behavior for treatment is also important because of its repeated association in research with a variety of later maladjustments during the adolescent and young adult years (Olweus, 1979; Patterson, 1982; Patterson et al., 1992; Tremblay, Pihl, Vitaro, & Dobkin, 1994). That is, defiant and coercive behavior, especially if it is of such magnitude and duration that it leads to referral for mental health services, is also a precursor or link to the development of other, more serious forms of antisocial behavior, criminal activity, and substance abuse (Barkley, Fischer, Edelbrock, & Smallish, 1990; Lahey & Loeber, 1994; Loeber, 1990; Lynskey & Fergusson, 1994; Patterson, 1982; Patterson et al., 1992). This can be seen in Table 1.5 where the ages of onset of various disruptive behaviors are shown. The pattern here is obvious; there is a developmental staging in the relationship of oppositional child behavior to later stages of physical aggression, status offenses, and crimes against property (Frick et al., 1993; Loeber, 1988, 1990; Loeber et al., 1992). Childhood oppositional behavior also significantly predicts later problems with academic performance and peer acceptance (Hinshaw & Anderson, 1996; Loeber, 1990; Patterson, 1982; Patterson et al., 1992; Tremblay et al., 1992; Wells & Forehand, 1985). The risk for later depression, suicidal ideation, and suicide attempts is also greater in children with defiant or aggressive behavior (Capaldi, 1992; Patterson, 1982; Patterson et al., 1992; Wenning, Nathan, & King, 1993). Thus, research is coming to show that the presence of oppositional defiant behavior, or social aggression, in children is the most highly stable of childhood psychopathologies over development and is a more significant predictor of a widespread array of negative social and academic risks than are most other forms of deviant child behavior (Farrington, 1995; Hinshaw & Anderson, 1996; Loeber, 1988, 1990; Fischer et al., 1993; Olweus, 1979, 1980; Paternite & Loney, 1980; Patterson, 1982;

TABLE 1.5. Median Age of Onset Reported by Parent of Symptoms of ODD and CD as a Function of the Quadrants Displayed in Figure 1.1

Median age (years)	D: Oppositional	B: Aggression	A: Property	C: Status
4.0	Stubborn			
5.0	Loses temper			
6.0	Defies, argues, touchy	Spiteful, fights, blames others		
6.5	Annoys others		Lies, hurts animals	
7.0	Angry	Bullies, cruel	Vandalizes	
7.5		Assaults	Steals	
8.0			Sets fires	
8.5				Truant
9.0				Swears
10.0				Runs away
Median of quadrant	6.0 years	6.75 years	7.25 years	9.0 years

Note. Adapted from Frick et al. (1993, p. 330). Copyright 1993 by Pergamon Press. Adapted by permission.

Patterson et al., 1992). These developmental risks become even more likely and more adverse when childhood defiant behavior is combined with higher levels of ADHD symptoms, particularly childhood impulsivity (Farrington, 1995; Hinshaw, 1987; Hinshaw & Anderson, 1996; Loeber, 1990; Moffitt, 1990; Olson, 1992; Tremblay et al., 1994). Oppositional behavior is therefore singled out for treatment because of the significant potential it carries for future negative consequences for the child if left untreated.

A Prelude to Effective Treatment of Other Problems

Finally, it would be hard to undertake the treatment of any other presenting problems of a child without first addressing the child's noncompliance. For example, attempting to toilet train a 3-year-old noncompliant child is not likely to prove successful until the child is taught to comply with requests. Similarly, parental tutoring of a school-age child during homework performance is also likely to fail as a consequence of the child's reliance on defiant behavior during work-related interactions with the parent. This will also be true of noncompliant children who must adhere to other medical regimens or educational programs in that such programs will likely prove less successful until the child's compliance with adult instructions is developed.

Important Aspects of Deviant Parent–Child Interactions

The substantial body of research that exists on the parent–child relations in families with behavior problem children is too voluminous to review here. At the very least, interested readers should peruse the texts by Patterson (1982; Patterson et al., 1992) and the reviews by Hinshaw and Anderson (1996), Lahey and Loeber (1994), Loeber (1988, 1990), Forehand and McMahon (1981), and Wahler (1975). The more consistent and general findings from this research are important to consider in the clinical training of these families. I summarize them briefly below.

Without a doubt, research repeatedly demonstrates that the quality or nature of parent–child interactions is strongly and reliably associated with childhood noncompliant, defiant, and aggressive behavior patterns, and the persistence of these behaviors over development, as well as the risk for later adolescent delinquency (Farrington, 1995; Haapasalo & Tremblay, 1994; Lahey & Loeber, 1994; Loeber, 1988, 1990; Patterson, 1982; Patterson et al., 1992; Schachar & Wachsmuth, 1990). Children with oppositional behavior show a poorer quality of attachment relationships to their parents (Speltz, DeKlyen, Greenberg, & Dryden, 1995). The parents of such children also provide highly inconsistent and, at times, even positive consequences to children for their deviant behavior (Dumas & Wahler, 1985; Patterson, 1982). Such poor attachment, unpredictable consequation, and even inadvertent reinforcement of defiant behavior may serve to increase and sustain occurrences of oppositional child behavior in future interactions. When children act out, throw temper tantrums, or directly oppose commands, it is surely difficult not to attend to such behavior. Even though such attention may seem negative to the parents, it may still serve to increase future oppositional behavior (Dumas & Wahler, 1985; Snyder & Brown, 1983). On other occasions, parents may provide positive attention or rewards to children in an effort to get them to stop "making a scene," such as in a store, restaurant, or other public place. Buying a child the candy bar for which he has been throwing a tantrum is but one obvious way in which parents may accelerate the acquisition and maintenance of deviant child behavior.

Conversely, parents may also provide less attention or reinforcement to prosocial or appropriate behaviors of the child. Clinical experience suggests that parents of behavior problem children may monitor or survey child behaviors less often than in families of normal children, such that they may not always be aware of ongoing appropriate child behaviors (Loeber, 1990; Patterson, 1982). Even if they are aware that the child is behaving well, they may elect not to attend to the child or praise him for several reasons. One is that many parents report that when they praise or attend to good behavior in their child it only serves to provoke a burst of negative behavior from the child. This leads the parent to adopt the attitude of "let sleeping dogs lie" when they encounter ongoing acceptable child behavior. Research has not established that this reaction occurs when parents have tried to praise a behavior problem child or, if it does, what the learning history was that established this behavioral pattern. It is possible that parental praise for good behavior in a child prompts the child to misbehave because the child continues to receive parental attention if he/she does so. Had the child continued to behave well, the parent might have terminated the interaction, moving on to do something else. Another reason parents may fail to react positively when a defiant child behaves well is that parents dislike interacting with the problematic child and will choose to avoid interacting with the child when possible. Parents of chronically defiant children often develop animosity or "grudges" toward the child such that they will elect not to praise him when the child finally behaves well. This may eventually lead to parents spending significantly less leisure and recreational time with the defiant child simply because it is not fun to do so.

In addition, it is possible that parents of oppositional children, especially those children at risk for later delinquency, may monitor their children's activities less often (Haapasalo & Tremblay, 1994; Patterson, 1982; Patterson et al., 1992) and attend less to unacceptable behavior so as to avoid further confrontations with the child. As in the saying "out of sight, out of mind," parents may eventually reduce the amount of effort they expend monitoring a child's ongoing behavior within the home so as not to have to confront any minor unacceptable behavior that may be occurring. By overlooking the problem behavior, they do not have to face the aversiveness of another negative, coercive exchange with the child about the matter. This may explain the frequent clinical observation that some parents seem to be oblivious to ongoing negative behavior occurring in their presence—behavior other parents would normally react to in a corrective fashion. For whatever reason, some parents of oppositional children are simply not as invested in serving in parental roles to these children, possibly because of their own frequently younger-than-normal age when becoming parents, their social immaturity or limited intelligence, and even their own psychological or psychiatric disorders. Regardless of its origins, such a decline in parental monitoring and management of child conduct is associated with the development of some of the most serious forms of CD, which involve both covert antisocial behavior—such as lying, stealing, destruction of community property, and so forth—as well as overt antisocial acts, such as physical aggression toward others (Hinshaw & Anderson, 1996; Frick et al., 1993; Loeber, 1990; Loeber et al., 1993; Patterson, 1982; Patterson et al., 1992, 1993).

Parents may also be observed actually to punish prosocial or appropriate behavior at times, again because of possible resentment that may have developed over years of negative interactions with the child. Parents may often give "back-handed compliments" to a child for finally doing something correctly, as when they sarcastically remark, "It's about time you cleaned your room; why couldn't you do that yesterday?" For all of these reasons, parents are simply not providing appropriate consequences for ongoing child behavior that would be expected to manage or control it effectively.

This inconsistent and unpredictable punishing of both prosocial and antisocial child behavior, as well as intermittently and unpredictably rewarding both classes of child behavior, has been referred to as "indiscriminant" parenting, where the children are damned if they do and damned if they don't comply (Dumas & Wahler, 1985). Dumas and Wahler (1985) have hypothesized that this form of indiscriminant use of consequences by parents creates a great deal of social unpredictability within families and especially in the parent–child relationship. Such environments are experienced by both humans and animals as inherently aversive. Any response by the child in such a situation that may be instrumental in reducing unpredictability will be negatively reinforced for doing so and thereby increase in frequency. Thus, children may emit various forms of defiant and aggressive behavior toward parents, based on which of these forms increases predictability in the course of parent–child interactions.

In a somewhat related theory also involving negative reinforcement, Patterson (1976, 1982) has argued that both parents and children in families with behavior disordered children are negatively reinforced for behaving in aggressive and coercive ways toward each other. Substantial research supports this argument (Patterson, 1982; Patterson et al., 1992, 1993; Snyder & Patterson, 1995). In this theory, the negative behavior of one member of the parent–child dyad serves to terminate the ongoing negative behavior of the other, thereby negatively reinforcing the first member's "coercive" behavior. He proposes that this may explain why parents and children, once having begun a negative interaction with each other, will escalate their negative behavior toward each other very quickly to intense levels of aggression or coercion. Furthermore, the likelihood that such forms of interaction will occur again is greatly increased as a result (Snyder & Patterson, 1995).

To appreciate the substantial clinical implications of this theory, it is first necessary to remember that negative reinforcement is *not* the same as punishment—a mistake often made by those less experienced in behavioral terminology. Negative reinforcement is said to occur when, during a situation where the child is subjected to aversive, unpleasant, or otherwise negative stimuli, the child emits a behavior that successfully terminates the ongoing aversive situation or permits him to escape from future such situations. For instance, when the parent attempts to impose the command of getting ready for bed while the child is watching a favorite television program, the child often finds this imposition to be aversive. The child may oppose, resist, or otherwise escape from the parental demand through defiant, aggressive, or other coercive behavior that delays having to get ready for bed. The child's success at escaping from the command, even if only temporarily, negatively reinforces his/her oppositional behavior. The next time the parent asks the child to get ready for bed, the likelihood of the child resisting the command has increased. The more a parent persists at repeating the request, the more intense the child's resistance may become due to this previous success at escaping or avoiding the activity specified in the command. As already noted above, many parents may eventually acquiesce to this type of coercive behavior. Parents need not acquiesce to every command for a child to acquire resistant behavior.

However, parents may also acquire aggressive or coercive behavior toward their defiant child by much the same process. In this case, the parent may have been successful on occasion at getting a child to cease whining, refusing, or tantruming and to comply with a command through the parent's use of yelling, screaming, or even physical aggression against the child. The parent may also have discovered that rapidly increasing the intensity of his/her negative behavior toward the child is more successful at getting the child to capitulate and obey, especially if the child initially opposes the command. Hence, in subsequent situations the parent may escalate very quickly to intense negative behavior toward a child due to a previous history of success at terminating oppositional child behavior by this means. The parent need not be successful with this strategy every time or even the majority of times the parent confronts oppositional behavior in order to maintain this type of parental behavior across most command–compliance encounters with the defiant child. Only occasional success with coercive behavior is needed to sustain this type of behavior in parents.

Viewed from this perspective, both parent and child have a prior history of periodic but only partial success at escaping or avoiding each other's escalating aversive or coercive behavior. As a result, each will continue to employ it with the other in most command–compliance interactions. Over time, each learns that when a command–compliance situation arises, the faster each escalates his/her own negative emotional intensity and coerciveness, the more likely the other is to acquiesce to his/her demands. As a result, confrontational interactions between parent and child may escalate quickly to quite intense, emotional, and even aggressive confrontations, which, on some occasions, may end with physical abuse of the child by the parent, destruction of property by the child, assault by the child against the parent, or even self-injury by some children.

This view also implies that much deviant child behavior is not sustained by positive attention or reinforcement from the parent but by negative reinforcement (Patterson, 1982; Snyder & Brown, 1983). Accordingly, when a clinician tells such a parent to ignore deviant child behavior, it may only worsen the problem as it is likely to be viewed by the child as acquiescence. In many cases, parents cannot ignore the child because in so doing the child escapes from performing the command given by the parent. Parents in such a situation will have to continue interacting with the child if they wish to get the task accomplished. Many experienced clinicians have noted this problem in training parents of behavior problem children—ignoring deviant behavior is not always successful or even possible. Instead, a great deal of negative child behavior is developed through escape/avoidance learning (negative reinforcement) and is maintained because of its success in avoiding unpleasant activities often invoked by parents. As Patterson suggests, and as this program teaches, the parent training program must incorporate mild *and consistent* punishment (usually time out from reinforcement), as well as prevention of the child from escaping the parental command, if the program is to be successful at diminishing child noncompliance developed through negative reinforcement.

Patterson has also noted (1976, 1982) that parents are likely, once trained, to rely predominantly on the punishment methods taught in the program and to diminish their use of positive reinforcement methods over time. Therapists must anticipate this parental drift and regression and address it during the last few sessions of parent training as well as during follow-up booster sessions. Parents must be instructed that most punishment methods lose their effectiveness when relied on as the primary management technique with children. Without sufficient positive reinforcement methods being provided for the alternative, appropriate behavior desired from the child, such desirable behavior is unlikely to be maintained (see Shriver & Allen, 1996, for a discussion of similar problems in classroom management).

This review of several important aspects of deviant parent–child interactions has a number of implications for the training of such parents in effective child management procedures, the most important of which are that parents must be trained to (1) increase the value of their attention generally, and its particular worth in motivating and reinforcing their child's positive behavior; (2) increase the positive attention and incentives they provide for compliance while decreasing the inadvertent punishment they provide for occasional compliance; (3) decrease the amount of inadvertent positive attention they provide to negative child behavior; (4) increase the use of immediate and consistent mild punishment for occurrences of child noncompliance; (5) ensure that escape from the activity being imposed upon the child does not occur (i.e., the command is eventually complied with by the child); (6) reduce the frequency of repeat commands parents employ so as to avoid delays to consequences (act, don't yak); (7) recognize and rapidly terminate escalating and confrontive negative interactions with the child; and (8) ensure that the parents do not regress to a predominantly punitive child management strategy once training has been completed. All of this, then, should serve to reduce the unpredictability involved in indiscriminant parenting while ensuring that child coercive behaviors are unsuccessful in their function to escape or avoid parental requests, demands, and commands.

Causes of Noncompliance/Defiance in Children

Parent–Child Relationship

As discussed above, one of the major causes of noncompliance, defiance, and social aggression repeatedly identified in research studies is poor, ineffective, inconsistent, and indiscriminant child management methods being employed by parents, often combined with unusually harsh but inconsistent disciplinary methods and poor monitoring of child activities (Farrington, 1995; Loeber, 1990; Olweus, 1980; Patterson, 1982; Patterson et al., 1992). As a result, noncompliance and defiance by children become very effective methods for escaping or avoiding unpleasant, boring, or effortful tasks, perhaps increasing the predictability of consequences in parent–child exchanges (no matter how negative), and on some occasions even obtaining rewards by the child for doing so (e.g., candy for the tantrum in the store). But it would be erroneous to conclude from this that all noncompliant or defiant behavior is simply learned out of the parent–child relationship. Whereas the exact form, nature, or topography of the noncompliant and defiant responses and even their severity in a child probably have much to do with the child's learning history within a family, the probability of acquiring or emitting oppositional or noncompliant behavior is also affected by at least three other domains of influence (Loeber, 1990; Patterson, 1982). Combined with impaired child and family management practices (first factor), these three other causal influences make up a Four-Factor Model of oppositional behavior in children.

Child Characteristics

The second factor addresses the growing realization that children having certain temperaments and cognitive characteristics are more prone to emit coercive–aggressive behavior and acquire noncompliance than are other children. In particular, children who are easily prone to emotional responses (high emotionality), are often irritable, have poor habit regulation, are highly active, and/or are more inattentive and impulsive appear more likely to display disruptive behavior disorders and, therefore, to demonstrate defiant and coercive behavior than are children not having such negative temperamental characteristics (Loeber, 1988, 1990; Olweus, 1980; Patterson, 1982; Prior, 1992; Tschann, Kaiser, Chesney, Alkon, & Boyce, 1996). And although parental psychopathology and poor marital and family functioning may further exacerbate the risks of such children for greater defiance and aggression, negative temperamental features of the child are among the strongest influences in this process (Olweus, 1980) and may be sufficient in themselves to create these risks (Tschann et al., 1996). The effects of early childhood temperament may be gender specific: More negative temperament in infant and toddler boys may be predictive of higher risk for later oppositional behavior; in contrast, for toddler girls early negative temperament may predict a *decrease* in the risk for later aggressive behavior but possibly an increase in later risk for internalizing disorders (Keenan & Shaw, 1994; Shaw & Vondra, 1995).

Symptoms of ADHD, such as overactivity, inattention, and impulsivity, are typically considered aspects of temperament when studied in infants and toddlers. Should they persist into later preschool years and eventually school age, such symptoms are more likely to create parent–child interaction conflicts (Barkley, 1985; Barkley, Fischer, Edelbrock & Smallish, 1991; Danforth, Barkley, & Stokes, 1991; Fletcher, Fischer, Barkley, & Smallish, 1996; Johnston, 1996; Mash & Johnston, 1982). Symptoms of ADHD may prevent a child from finishing assigned activities and thus the child may be more likely to elicit increased commands, supervision, and negative reactions from parents. Children with higher levels of ADHD symptoms may also be more likely to respond to these reprimands and parental confrontations with negative emotional reactions. If such reactions result in the child's escaping further demands, according to the above theories of defiance, their use during subsequent commands by parents will be increased and sustained. The co-occurrence of ADHD symptoms, particularly that of poor impulse control, with early oppositional behavior is particularly virulent, predicting significantly greater family conflicts (Barkley, Anastopoulos, Guevremont, & Fletcher, 1992; Fletcher et al., 1996; Johnston, 1996) and worse developmental outcomes, particularly in the realm of later antisocial activity, than does either dimension of behavior alone (Hinshaw, 1987; Loeber, 1990; Moffitt, 1990; Tremblay et al., 1994).

Parent Characteristics

Noncompliance or defiance in children may also increase in probability as a result of a third factor, that is, similar temperamental and cognitive characteristics in the child's parents (Frick et al., 1992; Patterson, 1982). Immature, inexperienced, impulsive, inattentive, depressed, hostile, rejecting, or otherwise negatively temperamental parents are more likely to have defiant and aggressive children (Olweus, 1980; Patterson, 1982). This may be because they display poor attentional and monitoring abilities, inconsistent management strategies, and greater irritability and hostility toward their children, and provide less reinforcement for prosocial behavior (Barkley, Anastopoulos, et al., 1992; Dumas, Gibson, & Albin, 1989; Hops et al., 1987; Mann & MacKenzie, 1996). Through such inconsistent and indiscriminant parenting, then, children experience periodic success at avoiding demands, further reinforcing the children's use of oppositional or coercive behavior. Such increases in child coercive behavior may then feed back further to affect detrimentally parent mood, sense of competence, self-esteem, and even marital functioning in a vicious, reciprocal cycle of bidirectional effects. Such parents may also employ coercive behavior with others in the family, providing a model of such behavior for the child to imitate (Patterson, 1982). In particular, the level of maternal depression and maternal and paternal psychopathology, especially antisocial personality disorder or criminality, are significantly associated with risk for childhood oppositional and aggressive behavior and later delinquency (Farrington, 1995; Frick et al., 1992; Keenan & Shaw, 1994; Olweus, 1980; Schachar & Wachsmuth, 1990). For these reasons and those noted below for stress events, parent psychological status must be a formal focus of the evaluation of children referred for defiant behavior (as will be discussed in Chapter 2).

Contextual Factors

The fourth factor involves larger contextual events surrounding the family, both internal and external to it, which may create or contribute to increased risks for child defiant behavior and aggression as well as later delinquency (Mann & MacKenzie, 1996; Patterson, 1982; Tschann et al., 1996; Wahler & Graves, 1983). As noted earlier, maternal social isolation is one such factor (Wahler, 1980), as is maternal marital status. Single mothers are the most likely to have significantly aggressive children, followed by mothers who live with male partners but are unmarried. Married mothers have the lowest rates of aggressive children, with these associations being moderated somewhat by higher social class (Pearson, Ialongo, Hunter, & Kellam, 1993; Vaden-Kiernan, Ialongo, Pearson, & Kellam, 1995). Marital discord also has been repeatedly linked to child disruptive and defiant behavior (Patterson, 1982; Schachar & Wachsmuth, 1990), although debate continues over the mechanisms involved in this relationship. Also noted earlier, family social disadvantage or social adversity is another factor associated with risks for childhood defiant and aggressive behavior (Farrington, 1995; Haapasalo & Tremblay, 1994; Patterson, 1982; Patterson et al., 1992). These stress events or settings appear to act on child misbehavior via their influence on creating inconsistency, indiscriminacy, inattention, and parental irritability in child management methods by parents. Such parental behavior further predisposes children to develop or sustain noncompliance or defiance within family interactions.

The relationships among the third and fourth factors above and child defiant behavior are nicely illustrated in Figure 1.4, drawn from Patterson's programmatic research on aggressive children and their families. As noted above, circumstances both internal and external to the family may contribute directly to child antisocial behavior but also make indirect contributions in many cases through their impact on the child and even family management practices of the parents. Notice also that for some of these circumstances, a reciprocal relationship exists wherein they may contribute to antisocial behavior in a child but such behavior, once developed, contributes to a worsening of these circumstances, such as in marital conflict, divorce, and parent psychiatric disturbances. Although not shown in this diagram, more recent research with ADHD children suggests that disruptive and oppositional behavior may feed back to increase parental alcohol use as well (Pelham & Lang, 1993).

It is all too common for clinicians to observe that many families referred for treatment of a defiant child have most or all of these predisposing characteristics: temperamental, im-

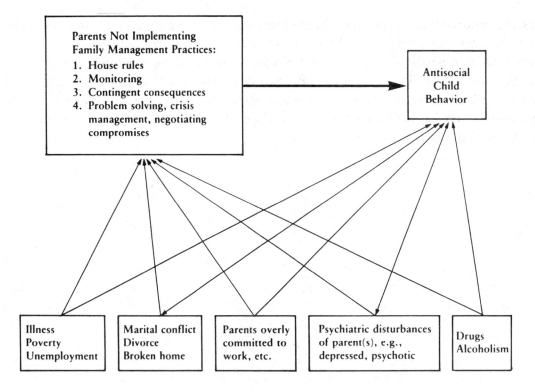

FIGURE 1.4. The relations among family management practices, crises, and antisocial child behavior. From Patterson (1982, p. 217). Copyright 1982 by Castalia Publishing Co. Reprinted by permission.

pulsive, active, and inattentive children being raised by immature, temperamental, and impulsive parents within a family experiencing greater marital, financial, health, and personal distress in its members, where management of the child is characterized by inconsistent, harsh, indiscriminant, and coercive parenting often along with reduced parental monitoring of the child's activities.

Summary

This chapter has described the importance of focusing on child noncompliance and defiance as the major target of the parent training program to be presented here. The processes whereby children may develop, maintain, or increase their rate of oppositional, defiant, or noncompliant behavior were discussed in some detail, and it appears that such behavior is chiefly sustained by its success at terminating parental demands and enabling the child to escape or avoid generally unpleasant, effortful, or boring tasks assigned by parents, while permitting the child to continue in a previous, more desirable activity. It was shown that parents may also come to escalate their own negative behavior toward the child because such behavior occasionally succeeds at terminating ongoing unpleasant child behavior, such as tantrums or defiance, and getting eventual child compliance. Both parents and children may be more predisposed toward such types of coercive behavior by virtue of their particular profile of temperamental patterns and psychological disorders. Larger contextual events such as stress, marital discord, parental social isolation, or events impacting the family from outside may serve to increase the probability of defiant child behavior by virtue of the toll these events take on the consistency of parental management of the child, the positive reinforcement of compliant child behavior, and the general monitoring of child activities by parents.

CHAPTER 2

Clinical Assessment of Defiant Children

It is not the intent here to provide a detailed review of the manner in which a thorough clinical evaluation should be conducted with behavior problem children and their families. Instead, this section will highlight the major topics that should be covered and several methods that may be used in evaluating oppositional children and their parents. Many such methods exist. Only that approach recommended by the author will receive emphasis here. Other methods are discussed in the texts by Mash and Terdal (1997), Barkley (1990), and Forehand and McMahon (1981), among others.

Assessment Issues

The evaluation of defiant children incorporates multiple assessment methods relying on several informants concerning the nature of the children's difficulties (and strengths!) across multiple situations. To accomplish this, parent, child, and teacher interviews are conducted, parent and teacher rating scales of child behavior and rating scales or surveys of child adaptive functioning should be obtained, and parent self-report measures of relevant psychiatric conditions and of parent and family functioning also should be collected. Some clinicians may wish to collect laboratory measures of ADHD symptoms, if that disorder is present, as well as direct observations of parent–child interactions. And, of course, children in whom intellectual or developmental delays or learning disabilities are suspected should receive psychological testing of these domains if such has not already been performed.

There are several goals to bear in mind in the evaluation of children for defiant behavior. A major goal of such an assessment is not only the determination of the presence or absence of psychiatric disorders, such as ODD, CD, and/or ADHD, but also the differential diagnosis of ODD from other childhood psychiatric disorders. This requires extensive clinical knowledge of these other psychiatric disorders, and the reader is referred to Mash and Barkley's (1996) text on child psychopathology for a review of the major childhood disorders. In evaluating defiant children, it may be necessary to draw on measures that are normed for the individual's ethnic background, if such instruments are available, so as to preclude the overdiagnosis of minority children when diagnostic criteria developed from white children are extrapolated to them.

A second purpose of the evaluation is to begin delineating the types of interventions that will be needed to address the psychiatric disorders and psychological, academic, and social impairments identified in the course of assessment. As noted later, these interventions may include individual counseling, parent training in behavior management, family therapy, classroom behavior modification, psychiatric medications, and formal special educational services, to name just a few. For a more thorough discussion of treatments for childhood disorders, the reader is referred to Mash and Barkley (in press).

Another important purpose of the evaluation is the determination of comorbid conditions and whether or not these may affect prognosis or treatment decision making. For instance, the presence of high levels of physically assaultive behavior by the child may signal that a parent training program such as this may be contraindicated, at least for the time being, because of its likelihood of temporarily increasing child violence toward parents when limits on noncompliance with parental commands are established. Or consider the presence of high levels of anxiety specifically and internalizing symptoms more generally in children with ODD who may have ADHD as well. Research has shown such symptoms to be a predictor of poorer responses to stimulant medication (DuPaul, Barkley, & McMurray, 1994). Similarly, the presence of high levels of irritable mood, severely hostile and defiant behavior, and periodic episodes of serious physical aggression and destructive behavior may be early markers for later Bipolar Disorder (manic depression) in children. Oppositional behavior is almost universal in juvenile-onset Bipolar Disorder (Wozniak & Biederman, 1995). Such a disorder will likely require the use of psychiatric medications in conjunction with a parent training program.

A further objective of the evaluation is to identify the pattern of the child's psychological strengths and weaknesses and to consider how these may affect treatment planning. This may also include gaining an impression of the parents' own abilities to carry out the treatment program, as well as the family's social and economic circumstances and the treatment resources that may (or may not) be available within their community and cultural group. Some determination will also need to be made as to the child's eligibility for special educational services within his/her school district, if eligible disorders, such as developmental delay, learning disabilities, or ADHD, are present.

As the foregoing discussion illustrates, the evaluation of a child for the presence of defiant behavior is but one of many purposes of the clinical evaluation of ODD children. A brief discussion now follows of the different methods of assessment that may be used in the evaluation of defiant children.

Assessment Methods

Prior to the Evaluation

When parents call my clinic for an evaluation, a form is completed by the receptionist that gathers important demographic information about the child and parents, the reason for the referral, and insurance information that will be cross-checked with the insurance company, where necessary. This form is then reviewed by the billing agent for our clinic and the clinician who will receive this case. Depending on the clinician's area of specialization, some types of referrals may be inappropriate for the clinician's practice and can be screened out at this time for referral to more appropriate services.

It is the practice at our clinic to send out a packet of questionnaires to parents and teachers following the parents' call to the clinic but in advance of the scheduled appointment. In fact, the parents of children referred to our clinic will not be given an appointment date until these packets of information are completed and returned to the clinic. This assures that the packets will be completed reasonably promptly and that the information is available for review by the clinician prior to meeting with the family, making the evaluation process far more efficient in its collection of important information. In these days of increasing cost consciousness concerning mental health evaluations, particularly in managed care environments, the efficiency of the evaluation is paramount and time spent directly with the family is often limited and at a premium. This packet of information for the parents will include a form cover letter from the professional asking them to complete the packet of information and informing them that the appointment date will be given when this packet is returned. The packet also contains the General Instructions sheet, a Child and Family Information Form, and a Developmental and Medical History Form, all of which are provided in Part III of this manual. These forms and the others provided in Part III are available in Spanish from the publisher. In addition, the packet includes a reasonably comprehensive child behavior rating scale that covers the major dimensions of child psychopathology, such as the Child Behavior Checklist (CBCL; Achenbach & Edelbrock, 1983) or the Behavioral Assessment System for Children (BASC; Reynolds & Kamphaus, 1994). Also in this packet is a copy of the Disruptive Behavior Disorders Rating Scale (DBDRS), provided in Part III. This scale permits the clinician to obtain information ahead of the appointment concerning the presence of symptoms of ODD, CD, and ADHD and their severity; these disorders are quite common among children referred for defiant behavior. Clinicians wishing to assess adaptive behavior via the use of a questionnaire might consider including in this packet the Normative Adaptive Behavior Checklist (NABC; Adams, 1984) rather than administering the more time-consuming interview with the Vineland Adaptive Behavior Scale (Sparrow, Baila, & Cicchetti, 1984) during the family's appointment. Finally, parents are sent the Home Situations Questionnaire (HSQ; also provided in Part III) in this packet so as to give the clinician a quick appreciation for the pervasiveness and severity of the child's disruptive behavior across a variety of home and public situations. Such information will be of clinical interest not only for indications of pervasiveness and severity of behavior problems, but also for focusing discussions around these situations during the evaluation and subsequent parent training program. These rating scales are discussed below.

A similar packet of information is sent to the child's teachers, with parental written permission obtained beforehand, of course. This packet does not contain the Developmental and Medical History Form or any adaptive behavior survey that may have been included for parents. This packet would contain the teacher version of the CBCL or BASC, the School Situations Questionnaire (SSQ; Barkley, 1987, 1990; see Part III), and the DBDRS. The Social Skills Rating Scale (Gresham & Elliott, 1990) may also be included and can be informative about the child's social problems in school as well as academic competence, as quickly screened by this relatively brief scale. If possible, it is quite useful to contact the child's teachers by telephone for a brief interview prior to meeting with the family. Otherwise, this can be done following the family's appointment.

Once the parent and teacher packets have been returned, the family should be contacted by telephone and given their appointment. It is also our custom to send out a letter confirming this appointment date, with directions for driving to the clinic. With this letter can be sent a detailed instruction sheet entitled "How to Prepare for Your Child's Evaluation," which is provided in Part III (Form 8). This gives the family some information about what to expect on the day of the evaluation and may set them at ease if having a mental health evaluation is disconcerting or anxiety inducing for them.

This preparation leaves the following to be done on the day of the appointment: (1) parental and child interview, (2) completion of self-report rating scales by the parents, and (3) any psychological testing that may be indicated by the nature of the referral (e.g., intelligence and achievement testing, etc.).

Parental Interview

Although often criticized for its unreliability and subjectivity, the parental (often maternal) interview remains an indispensable part of the clinical assessment of children. If one were limited to just a single method for psychological evaluation of a child, the parental (maternal) interview, unhesitatingly, would be the method of choice. Whether wholly accurate or not, parental reports provide the most ecologically valid and important source of information concerning children's difficulties. It is frequently the parents' complaints that have led to the referral of the children, that will affect the parents' perceptions of and reactions to the children, and that will influence the parents' adherence to the treatment recommendations to be made. Moreover, the reliability and accuracy of the parental interview hinge on the manner in which it is conducted and the specificity of the questions posed by the interview. Diagnostic reliability is greatly enhanced by interviewing that utilizes highly specific questions about symptoms of psychopathology that have been empirically demonstrated to have a high degree of association with particular disorders. The interview must also focus on the specific complaints about the child's psychological adjustment and any functional parameters (eliciting and consequating events) associated with those problems, if psychosocial and educational treatment planning is to be based on the evaluation.

Demographic Information

If not obtained in advance, the routine demographic data concerning the child and family (e.g., ages of child and family members; child's date of birth; parents' names, addresses, employers, occupations, and religion(s); and the child's school, teachers, and physician) should be obtained at the outset of the appointment. I also use this initial introductory period as a time to review with the family any legal constraints on the confidentiality of information obtained during the interview, such as the clinician's legal duty (as required by state law) to report to state authorities instances of suspected child abuse, threats that the child (or parents) may make to cause physical harm to other specific individuals (the duty to inform), and threats that the child (or parents) may make to harm him/herself (e.g., suicide threats).

Major Parental Concerns

The interview then proceeds to the major referral concerns of the parents, and of the professional who referred the child where appropriate. An interview form I designed is provided in Part III (The Clinical Interview—Parent Report Form) and can be helpful in collecting the information discussed below. This form not only contains extensive sections for obtaining the important information discussed here, but also contains the diagnostic criteria used for ODD as well as the other childhood disorders most likely to be seen in conjunction with ODD (i.e., ADHD, CD, Anxiety and Mood Disorders, Bipolar Disorder). This form allows clinicians to collect the essential information likely to be of greatest value to them in evaluating defiant children, using a convenient and standardized format across their client populations.

General descriptions of concerns by parents must be followed with specific questions by the examiner to elucidate the details of the problems and any apparent precipitants that can be identified. Such an interview probes for not only the specific nature, frequency, age of onset, and chronicity of the problematic behaviors, but also for the situational and temporal variations in the behaviors and their consequences. If the problems are chronic, which they often are, determining what prompted the referral at this time reveals much about parental perceptions of the children's problems, current family circumstances related to the problems' severity, and parental motivation for treatment.

Review of Major Developmental Domains

Following this, one should review with the parents potential problems that might exist in the developmental domains of motor, language, intellectual, thinking, academic, emotional, and social functioning. Such information greatly aids in the differential diagnosis of the children's problems. To accomplish this requires that the examiner have an adequate knowledge of the diagnostic features of other childhood disorders, some of which may present as ODD. For instance many children with atypical Pervasive Developmental Disorders (Childhood Onset), Asperger's Disorder, or early Bipolar Disorder may be viewed by their parents as ODD or ADHD children, as the parents are more likely to have heard about the latter disorders than the former ones and will recognize some of the qualities in their children. Questions about inappropriate thinking, affect, social relations, and motor peculiarities may reveal a more seriously and pervasively disturbed child. If such symptoms seem to be present, the clinician may want to employ the Children's Atypical Development Scale (see Barkley, 1990) at this point, to obtain a more thorough review of these symptoms. Inquiry also must be made as to the presence or history of tics or Tourette's Disorder in the child or the immediate biological family members. Where noted, these would result in a recommendation either against the use of stimulant drugs in the treatment of a defiant child with comorbid ADHD or, at the very least, cautious use of low doses of such medicine to preclude the exacerbation of the child's tic disorder (DuPaul et al., 1994).

School, Family, and Treatment Histories

Information on the school and family histories should also be obtained, the latter of which includes a discussion of possible psychiatric difficulties in the parents and siblings, marital difficulties, and any family problems centered around chronic medical conditions, employment problems, or other potential stress events within the family. Of course, the examiner will want to obtain some information about prior treatments received by the children and their families for these presenting problems. Where the history suggests potentially treatable medical or neurological conditions (allergies, seizures, Tourette's Disorder, etc.), a referral to a physician is essential. Without evidence of such problems, however, referral to a physician for examination usually fails to reveal any further information of use in the treatment of the children. An exception to this is where use of psychiatric medications is contemplated, in which case a referral to a physician is clearly indicated.

Review of Childhood Disorders

As part of the general interview of the parent, the examiner will need to cover the symptoms of the major child psychiatric disorders likely to be seen in defiant children. These are set forth in the structured interview provided in Part III. But regardless of whether this particular interview method is employed, some review of the major childhood disorders in DSM-IV (American Psychiatric Association, 1994) in some semistructured or structured way is imperative if any semblance of a reliable and differential approach to diagnosis and the documentation of comorbid disorders is to occur. In using the interview in Part III for these purposes, care must be exercised in the evaluation of minority children so as not to overdiagnose psychiatric disorders in such children by virtue simply of differing cultural standards for child behavior. Recall the discussion in Chapter 1 about ensuring not only that the behaviors of children are statistically deviant, but that they also are associated with evidence of impairment in adaptive functioning or some other "harmful dysfunction." As one means of partially precluding overidentification of psychopathology in minority children, the following adjustment has been recommended. When reviewing the psychiatric symptoms for the childhood disorders with parents, should the parent indicate that a symptom is present, follow up with the question, "Do you consider this to be a problem for your child compared to other children of the same ethnic or minority group?" Only if the parent answers "yes" to this second question is the symptom to be considered present for purposes of psychiatric diagnosis.

When applying the diagnostic criteria for ODD (see Chapter 1, Table 1.2) to defiant children, several problems with the criteria should be borne in mind and adjustments made for them as needed:

1. The cutoff score on the symptom list (four of eight) was primarily developed on children ages 4–16 years. The extrapolation of these thresholds to age ranges outside of those in the field trial is questionable. Studies of large populations of children (Achenbach & Edelbrock, 1983, 1986) indicate that the behaviors associated with ODD tend to decline in frequency within the population over development. Thus, a somewhat higher threshold may be needed for preschool children (ages 2–4) if the same developmentally relative level of deviance (93rd percentile) is to be used to define the disorder.

2. The children used in the DSM-IV field trial for ODD and CD were predominantly males, by an average ratio of 3:1 (Lahey, Applegate, Barkley, et al., 1994). Studies of large samples of children reliably demonstrate that parents and teachers report lower levels of those behaviors associated with ODD in girls than in boys (Achenbach & Edelbrock, 1983, 1986; Goyette, Conners, & Ulrich, 1978). It is possible, then, that the cutoff point on the DSM-IV symptom lists for these disorders, based as they are mainly on males, are unfairly high for females. In other words, using current DSM-IV thresholds, a girl must meet a higher standard of deviance relative to girls than a boy must do relative to boys in order to be diagnosed as ODD or CD. The argument hinges on the critical point of whether such a girl demonstrates impairment despite having a lower level of symptoms than a boy; this point has not yet been adequately studied but others have made a similar argument based on the available research literature on gender differences in the nature of ODD and CD (Zoccolillo, 1993). In any case, clinicians should keep this point in mind as a girl who falls but a single symptom shy of the diagnostic cutoff score in DSM-IV for ODD and CD may well warrant the diagnosis nonetheless.

3. The criterion that duration of symptoms be at least 6 months was not specifically studied in the field trial and was held over from earlier DSMs primarily out of tradition. Symptoms of ODD are quite common during the preschool years and may persist for periods of 6 months or more without necessarily indicating the presence of a disorder in the child. Also, some research even suggests a large mi-

nority (25%) of children initially diagnosed with ODD will no longer qualify for the diagnosis when reevaluated a year later (see Chapter 1). Children whose symptoms persisted for at least a year or more, however, are likely to remain deviant in their behavior pattern into the elementary school years, suggesting that clinicians might want to adjust the duration criterion to 12 months.

Adjustments may also need to be made to the DSM-IV criteria for ADHD (Chapter 1, Table 1.4). Given the high probability of ADHD occurring in children diagnosed as ODD, these adjustments are listed below:

1. Again, the cutoff scores on both symptom lists (six of nine) were primarily developed on children ages 4–16 years in the DSM-IV field trial (Lahey, Applegate, McBurnett, et al., 1994), making the extrapolation of these thresholds to age ranges outside of those in the field trial of uncertain validity. ADHD behaviors tend to decline in frequency within the population over development, again suggesting that a somewhat higher threshold may be needed for preschool children (ages 2–4).

2. The children used in the DSM-IV field trial, as noted above, were predominantly males. Studies reliably demonstrate that parents and teachers report lower levels of those behaviors associated with ADHD in girls than in boys (Achenbach & Edelbrock, 1983, 1986; DuPaul, 1991). It is possible, then, that the cutoff points on the DSM-IV symptom lists, based as they are mainly on males, are unfairly high for females.

3. The specific age of onset of 7 years is not particularly critical for identifying ADHD children. The field trial for the DSM-IV found that ADHD children having various ages of onset were essentially similar in their nature and severity of impairments so long as their symptoms had developed prior to ages 10–12 years (Applegate et al., 1995). And so stipulating an onset of symptoms in childhood is probably sufficient for purposes of clinical diagnosis.

4. Once again, the criterion that duration of symptoms be at least 6 months was not specifically studied in the field trial and was held over from earlier DSMs primarily out of tradition. Some research on preschool children suggests that a large number of 2- to 3-year-olds may manifest the symptoms of ADHD as part of that developmental period and that they may remain present for periods of 3–6 months or longer (Campbell, 1990; Palfrey, Levine, Walker, & Sullivan, 1985). Children whose symptoms persisted for at least a year or more, however, were likely to remain deviant in their behavior pattern into the elementary school years (Campbell & Ewing, 1990; Palfrey et al., 1985). Adjusting the duration criterion to 12 months would seem to make good clinical sense.

5. The criterion that symptoms must be evident in at least two or more settings (e.g., home, school, work) essentially requires that children have sufficient symptoms of ADHD by both parent and teacher report before they can qualify for the diag-

nosis. This requirement bumps up against a methodological problem inherent in comparing parent and teacher reports. On average, the relationship of behavior ratings from these two sources tends to be fairly modest, averaging about 0.30 (Achenbach, McConaughy, & Howell, 1987). If parent and teacher ratings are unlikely to agree across various behavioral domains being rated, this sets unnecessary limits on the number of children qualifying for the diagnosis of ADHD, due mainly to measurement artifact. Fortunately, some evidence demonstrates that children who meet DSM criteria (in this case, DSM-III-R) by parent reports have a high probability of meeting the criteria by teacher reports (Biederman, Keenan, & Faraone, 1990). Even so, stipulating that parents and teachers *must* agree on the diagnostic criteria before a diagnosis can be rendered is probably unwise and unnecessarily restrictive. For now, clinicians are advised to seek evidence that the child's symptoms of the disorder have existed at some time in the past or present in several settings, rather than insisting on the agreement of the parents with a current teacher in order to grant the diagnosis.

The foregoing issues should be kept in mind when applying the DSM criteria to particular clinical cases. It helps if one appreciates the fact that the DSM represents guidelines for diagnosis, not rules of law or dogmatic "religious" proscriptions. Some clinical judgment is always going to be needed in the application of such guidelines to individual cases in clinical practice. For instance, if a child meets all criteria for ADHD including both parent and teacher agreement on symptoms except that the age of onset for the symptoms and impairment is 9 years, should the diagnosis be withheld? Given the above discussion concerning the lack of specificity for an age of onset of 7 years with ADHD, the wise clinician would grant the diagnosis anyway. Likewise, if an 8-year-old girl meets three of the eight ODD symptoms and all other conditions are met for ODD, the diagnosis should likely be granted, given the comments above about gender bias within these criteria. Some flexibility (and common sense!), then, must be incorporated into the clinical application of any DSM criteria.

For years, some clinicians have eschewed diagnosing children entirely, viewing it as a mechanistic and dehumanizing practice that merely results in unnecessary labeling of children. Moreover, they may feel that it gets in the way of appreciating the clinical uniqueness of each case, unnecessarily homogenizing the heterogeneity out of clinical cases. Some may have believed that labeling a child's condition with a diagnosis was unnecessary, as it was far more important, in planning behavioral treatments, to articulate the child's pattern of behavioral and developmental excesses and deficits than it was to give a diagnosis. Although there may have been some justification for these views in the past, particularly prior to the development of more empirically based diagnostic criteria, this is no longer the case in view of the wealth of research that went into creating the DSM-IV childhood disorders and their criteria. This is not to say that clinicians should not proceed to document patterns of behavioral deficits and excesses, as such documentation is important for treatment planning; only that this should not be used as an excuse to omit diagnosis. Furthermore, given that the protection of rights and access to educational and other services may actually hinge on the awarding or withholding of the diagnosis of ADHD, dispensing with diagnosis altogether could well be considered professional negligence. For these reasons, and others, clinicians must review in some systematic way with the parent of each referred child the symptom lists and other diagnostic criteria for various childhood mental disorders.

The parental interview may also reveal that one parent, usually the mother, has more difficulty managing the ODD child than the other. Care should be taken to discuss differences in the parents' approaches to management and any marital problems this may have spawned. Such difficulties in child management can often lead to reduced leisure and recreational time for the parents, and increased conflict within the marriage and often within the extended family, should relatives live nearby. It is often helpful to inquire as to what attributions the parents may have about the causes or origins of their child's behavioral difficulties as this may unveil areas of ignorance or misinformation that will require attention later during the initial counseling of the family about the child's disorder(s) and their likely causes. The examiner also should briefly inquire about the nature of parental and family social activities to determine how isolated, or insular, the parents are from the usual social support networks in which many parents are involved. Research by Wahler (1980), discussed in the Introduction and in Chapter 1, has shown that the degree of maternal insularity is significantly associated with failure in subsequent parent training programs. Where present to a significant degree, such a finding might auger for addressing the isolation as an initial goal of treatment rather than progressing directly to child behavior management training with that family.

The parental interview can then conclude with a discussion of the children's positive characteristics and attributes as well as potential rewards and reinforcers desired by the children that will prove useful in later parent training on contingency management methods. Some parents of ADHD children have had such chronic and pervasive management problems that upon initial questioning they may find it hard to report anything positive about their children. Getting them to begin thinking of such attributes is actually an initial step toward treatment, as the early phases of parent training will teach parents to focus on and attend to desirable child behaviors (Forehand & McMahon, 1981).

At a later appointment, perhaps even during the initial session of parent training, the examiner may wish to pursue more details about the nature of the parent–child interactions surrounding the following of rules by the child. Parents should be questioned about the child's ability to accomplish commands and requests in a satisfactory manner in various settings, to adhere to rules of conduct governing behavior in various situations, and to demonstrate self-control (rule following) appropriate to the child's age in the absence of adult supervision. To accomplish this, I have found it useful to follow the format set forth in Table 2.1, in which parents are questioned about their interactions with their children in a variety of home and public situations. Where problems are said to occur, the examiner follows up with the list of questions in Table 2.1. If the parents have completed the HSQ as part of this evaluation, then the responses on that questionnaire can be used as the starting point for this interview, following up each situation endorsed as a problem on that questionnaire with these same follow-up questions.

Such an approach yields a wealth of information on the nature of parent–child interactions across settings, the type of noncompliance shown by the child (e.g., stalling, starting the task but failing to finish it, outright opposition and defiance, etc.), the particular management style employed by parents to deal with noncompliance, and the particular types of coercive behaviors used by the child as part of the noncompliance. This may take 30–40 minutes beyond the parental interview described above but is well worth the time invested where it is possible to do so, especially if parent training in child behavior management is likely to be subsequently recommended for this family. When time constraints make this problematic, the HSQ rating scale that was developed to provide similar types of information can be used. After parents complete the scale, they can be questioned about one or two of the problem situations using the same follow-up questions as in Table 2.1. The HSQ scale is discussed below.

Child Interview

Some time should always be spent directly interacting with the referred child. The length of this interview depends on the age, intellectual level, and language abilities of the children. For preschool children, the interview may serve merely as a time to become acquainted with the child, noting his/her appearance, behavior, developmental characteristics, and general demeanor. For older children and adolescents, this time can be fruitfully spent

TABLE 2.1. Parental Interview Format for Assessing Child Behavior Problems at Home and in Public

Situations to be discussed	If a problem, follow-up questions to ask
Overall parent–child interactions	1. Is this a problem area? If so, then proceed with questions 2–9.
Playing alone	2. What does the child do in this situation that bothers you?
Playing with other children	3. What is your response likely to be?
Mealtimes	4. What will the child do in response to you?
Getting dressed/undressed	5. If the problem continues, what will you do next?
Washing and bathing	6. What is usually the outcome of this situation?
When parent is on telephone	7. How often do these problems occur in this situation?
When child is watching television	8. How do you feel about these problems?
When visitors are in your home	9. On a scale of 1 (no problem) to 9 (severe), how severe is this
When you are visiting someone else's home	problem for you?
In public places (stores, restaurants, church, etc.)	
When father is in the home	
When child is asked to do chores	
When child is asked to do school homework	
Bedtime	
When child is riding in the car	
When child is left with a babysitter	
Any other problem situations	

Note. From Barkley (1981, p. 98). Copyright 1981 by The Guilford Press. Reprinted by permission.

inquiring about the children's views of the reasons for the referral and evaluation, how they see the family functioning, any additional problems they feel they may have, how well they are performing at school, their degree of acceptance by peers and classmates, and what changes in the family they believe might make life for them happier at home. As with the parents, the children can be queried as to potential rewards and reinforcers they find desirable, which will prove useful in later contingency management programs.

Children below the age of 9–12 years are not especially reliable in their reports of their own disruptive behavior. The problem is compounded by the frequently diminished self-awareness and impulse control typical of defiant children with ADHD (Hinshaw, 1994). Such ODD/ADHD children often show little reflection about the examiner's questions and may lie or distort information in a more socially pleasing direction. Some will report they have many friends, have no interaction problems at home with their parents, and are doing well at school, in direct contrast with the extensive parental and teacher complaints of inappropriate behavior by these children. Because of this tendency of ADHD children to underreport the seriousness of their behavior, particularly in the realm of disruptive or externalizing behaviors (Barkley et al., 1991; Fischer et al., 1993), the diagnosis of ODD or ADHD is never based on the reports of the child. Nevertheless, children's reports of their internalizing symptoms, such as anxiety and depression, may be more reliable and so should play some role in the diagnosis of comorbid Anxiety or Mood Disorders in children with ADHD (Hinshaw, 1994).

Although noting the children's behavior, compliance, attention span, activity level, and impulse control within the clinic is useful, clinicians must guard against drawing any diagnostic conclusions from the cases where the children are not defiant in the clinic or office. Many ODD and ADHD children do not misbehave in clinicians' offices and so heavy reliance on such observations would clearly lead to false negatives in the diagnosis (Sleator & Ullmann, 1981). In some instances, the behavior of the children with their parents in the waiting area prior to the appointment may be a better indication of the children's management problems at home than is the children's behavior toward the clinician, particularly when this involves a one-to-one interaction between child and examiner.

This is not to say that office behavior of a child is entirely useless. Where it is grossly inappropriate or extreme, it may well signal the likelihood of problems in the child's natural settings, particularly school. It is the presence of relatively normal conduct by the child that may be an unreliable indicator of the child's normalcy elsewhere. For instance, in an ongoing study of 205 4- to 6-year-old children, I have examined the relationship of office behavior to parent and teacher ratings (Barkley, 1991). Of these children, 158 were identified at kindergarten registration as being 1.5 SD above the mean (93rd percentile) on parent ratings of ADHD and ODD (aggressive) symptoms. These children were subsequently evaluated for nearly 4 hours in a clinic setting, after which the examiner completed a rating scale of the child's behavior in the clinic. I then classified the children as falling below or above the 93rd percentile on these clinic ratings using data from a normal control group being tested as part of this project. The children were also classified as falling above or below this threshold on parent ratings of home behavior and teacher ratings of school behavior using the CBCL. I have found to date that there is no significant relationship between the children's clinic behavior (normal or abnormal) and the ratings by their parents. However, there is a significant relationship between abnormal ratings in the clinic and abnormal ratings by the teacher, in that 70% of the children classified as abnormal in their clinic behavior were also classified as such by the teacher ratings of class behavior, particularly on the externalizing behavior dimension. Normal behavior, however, was not necessarily predictive of normal behavior in either parent or teacher ratings. This suggests that abnormal or significantly disruptive behavior during a lengthy clinical evaluation may be a marker for similar behavioral difficulties in a school setting. Nevertheless, the wise clinician will contact the child's teacher directly to learn about the child's school adjustment rather than rely entirely on such inferences about school behavior from clinic office behavior.

Teacher Interview

At some point before or soon after the initial evaluation session with the family, contact with the children's teachers is essential so as to clarify further the nature of the children's problems. This will most likely be done by telephone unless the clinician works within the child's school system. Interviews with teachers have all of the same merits as do interviews with parents, providing a second ecologically valid source of indispensable information about the child's psychological adjustment, in this case, in the school setting. Like parent reports, teacher reports are also subject to bias, and the integrity of the reporter of information, be it parent or teacher, must always be weighed in judging the validity of the information itself.

Many defiant children, especially those with comorbid ADHD, have problems with academic performance and classroom behavior and the details of these difficulties need to be obtained. While this may initially be done by telephone, where time and resources permit a visit to the classroom and direct observation and recording of the children's behavior can prove quite useful if further documentation of comorbid ADHD behaviors is necessary for planning later contingency management programs for the classroom. Granted, this is unlikely to prove feasible for clinicians working outside of school systems, particularly in the climate of increasing managed health care plans that severely restrict the evaluation time that will be compensated. But for those professionals working within school systems, direct behavioral observations can prove very fruitful for diagnosis, and especially for treatment planning (Atkins & Pelham, 1992; DuPaul & Stoner, 1994).

Teachers should also be sent the rating scales mentioned above. These can be sent as a packet prior to the actual evaluation so that the results are available for discussion with the parents during the interview, as well as with the teacher during the subsequent telephone contact or school visit.

The teacher interview also should focus on the specific nature of the children's problems in the school environment, again following a behavioral format. The settings, nature, frequency, consequating events, and eliciting events of the major behavioral problems also can be explored. The follow-up questions used in the parental interview on parent–child interactions and shown in Table 2.1 may prove useful here as well. Teachers should be questioned about potential learning disabilities in the children, given the greater likelihood of occurrence of such disorders in this population. Where evidence suggests their existence, the evaluation of the children should be expanded to explore the nature and degree of such deficits as viewed by the teacher. Even where learning disabilities do not exist, defiant children having ADHD are more likely to have problems with sloppy handwriting, careless approaches to tasks, poor organization of their work materials, and academic underachievement relative to their tested abilities. Time should be taken with the teachers to explore the possibility of these problems.

Child Behavior Rating Scales for Parent and Teacher Reports

Child behavior checklists and rating scales have become an essential element in the evaluation and diagnosis of children with behavior problems. The availability of several scales with excellent normative data across a wide age range of children and having acceptable reliability and validity makes their incorporation into the assessment protocol quite convenient and extremely useful. Such information is invaluable in determining the statistical deviance of the children's problem behaviors and the degree to which other problems may be present. As a result, it is useful to mail a packet of these scales out to parents prior to the initial appointment asking that they be returned on or before the day of the evaluation, as described above. This permits the examiner to review and score them before interviewing the parents, allows for vague or significant answers to be elucidated in the interview, and serves to focus the subsequent interview on those areas of abnormality that may be highlighted in the responses to scale items.

Numerous child behavior rating scales exist, and the reader is referred to other reviews (Barkley, 1988, 1990) for greater details on the more commonly used scales and for a discussion of the requirements and underlying assumptions of behavior rating scales—assumptions that are all too easily overlooked in the clinical use of these instruments. Despite their limitations, behavior rating scales offer a means of gathering information from people who may have spent months or years with the child. Apart from interviews, there is no other means of obtaining such a wealth of information for so little investment of time. The fact that such scales provide a means of quantifying the opinions of others, often along qualitative dimensions, and of comparing these scores to norms collected on large groups of children are further merits of these instruments. Nevertheless, behavior rating scales are opinions and are subject to the oversights, prejudices, and limitations on reliability and validity such opinions may have.

Initially, it is advisable to utilize "broad-band" rating scales that provide coverage of the major dimensions of child psychopathology known to exist, such as depression, anxiety, withdrawal, aggression, delinquent conduct, and, of course, inattentive and hyperactive–impulsive behavior. These scales should be completed by parents and teachers. Such scales would be the BASC (Reynolds & Kamphaus, 1994) and the CBCL (Achenbach & Edelbrock, 1983), both of which have versions for parents and teachers and satisfactory normative information. (The CBCL can be obtained from Thomas Achenbach, PhD, Child and Adolescent Psychiatry, Department of Psychiatry, University of Vermont, 5 South Prospect St., Burlington, VT 05401. The BASC can be obtained from American Guidance Service, 4201 Woodland Rd., Circle Pines, MN 55014.)

The Personality Inventory for Children (Lachar, 1982) may also serve this purpose, provided that one of the shortened versions is employed for convenience and the more contemporary norms are used for scoring purposes. It is, however, a scale only for parents to complete, precluding the informative comparison that can (and should) be made between parent and teacher reports on the same scale. The original Conners Parent and Teacher Rating Scales (Conners, 1990) can also be used for this initial screening for psychopathology but they do not provide the breadth of coverage across all of these dimensions of psychopathology as do the aforementioned scales; this is particularly so for the revised versions of the Conners scales. The normative samples used for the Conners scales have been more limited than those for the CBCL and BASC, although this may be corrected by a new normative study now underway.

More narrow-band scales should also be employed in the initial screening of children that focus more specifically on the assessment of symptoms of ODD and ADHD. For this purpose, I have provided in Part III parent and teacher versions of the DBDRS, which obtains ratings of the DSM-IV symptoms of ODD, ADHD, and CD. To score the scale items related to ODD (Items 19–26), simply count the number of answers circled with a 2 or 3 as each of these is treated as a positively endorsed symptom of the disorder. Items with ratings of 0 or 1 are considered to be normal. If four or more items have been circled with answers of 2 or 3, this may indicate the presence of a clinical diagnosis of ODD, which should be corroborated through the parental interview form provided in Part III. For the ADHD symptom ratings, do very much the same thing. First count the number of items circled with a 2 or 3 for the Inattention items (Items 1–9). Then count the number of items answered this way for the Hyperactive–Impulsive items (Items 10–18). If at least six symptoms have been answered this way on either list, it is an indication that one of the ADHD subtypes may be present and should be corroborated through the clinical interview.

Norms have recently been collected by George DuPaul and colleagues at Lehigh University (Bethlehem, PA) for these ADHD items (DuPaul, Anastopoulos, et al., 1996; DuPaul, Power, et al., 1996). To score this rating scale, the clinician would want to add up *the total points* circled for all the items (including answers of 0's, and 1's) on the Inattention and Hyperactive–Impulsive lists separately. The 93rd percentile has typically been construed as reflecting clinical significance, and so below are listed the thresholds for the 93rd percentile for these scores for each of these lists, given separately by source of report, child age, and child gender:

Age (years)	Boys		Girls	
	Inattention	Hyperactive–Impulsive	Inattention	Hyperactive–Impulsive
		Parent ratings		
5–7	15	17	12	13
8–10	15	15	12	9
11–13	18.5	16	12.8	9
		Teacher ratings		
5–7	22	22	21	21.1
8–10	25	25	21	16.7
11–13	24	18	19	14.8

The remaining items 1–15 at the end of the Parent version of the DBDRS are for Conduct Disorder. Simply count the number of Yes answers and use the cutoff score from the DSM-IV for this disorder (see Table 1.3).

Another narrow-band scale specific to ADHD is the Child Attention Problems Scale, which has the advantage of being drawn directly from the teacher version of the CBCL and thus benefits from the rigor of standardization and norming that went into that scale's development (Achenbach & Edelbrock, 1986). Its disadvantage, like many of the specialized scales noted above, is that it does not employ the precise symptom lists for inattention and hyperactivity–impulsivity from the DSM-IV. Thus, high scores on this scale would not automatically indicate a diagnosis of ADHD to be granted just from the results of the scale alone. In fact, this is a good time to remind the reader that scores on rating scales, alone, are not sufficient to render a psychiatric diagnosis in a child, such as ODD or ADHD. This information must be combined with that obtained from the parent and teacher interviews, as well as the specialized knowledge of the clinician in differential diagnosis, before specific diagnoses in children should be rendered.

The pervasiveness of the child's behavior problems within the home and school settings should also be examined, as such measures of situational pervasiveness appear to have as much or more stability over time than do the aforementioned scales (Fischer et al., 1993). The HSQ and SSQ (Barkley, 1987, 1990) provide a means for doing so and normative information for these scales is available (Altepeter & Breen, 1992; Barkley, 1990; Barkley & Edelbrock, 1987; DuPaul & Barkley, 1992). The HSQ is provided in Part III and requires parents to rate their child's behavior problems across 16 different home and public situations. The SSQ, also provided in Part III, similarly obtains teacher reports of problems in 12 different school situations. Both scales are scored the same way to yield two separate scores. The first is the Number of Problem Settings, calculated simply by counting the number of items answered Yes. The second is the Mean Severity

Score calculated by summing the numbers circled beside the items and then dividing by the number of Yes answers. Again, using the 93rd percentile (1.5 *SD* above the mean) as an indication of clinical significance, scores at or above the following thresholds would be significant:

Age (years)	Boys		Girls	
	No. of problems	Severity	No. of problems	Severity
		Home ratings		
4–5	7.3	3.8	6.1	3.4
6–8	9.1	4.1	8.7	3.9
9–11	8.6	4.2	7.5	3.5
		School ratings		
6–8	7.4	4.5	4.0	3.1
9–11	7.6	5.1	4.5	2.6

Both the more specialized or narrow band scales focusing on symptoms of ODD and ADHD in the DBDRS, as well as the HSQ and SSQ can be used to monitor treatment response when given prior to and at the end of parent training in this program. They can also be used to monitor the behavioral effects of stimulant medication on children with ADHD. In that case, use of the Side Effects Rating Scale is also to be encouraged (see Barkley, 1990).

One of the most common problem areas for defiant children with comorbid ADHD is in their academic productivity. The amount of work typically accomplished by ADHD children at school is often substantially less than that done by their peers within the same period of time. Demonstrating such an impact of ADHD on school functioning is often critical for ADHD children to be eligible for special educational services (DuPaul & Stoner, 1994). The Academic Performance Rating Scale (see Barkley, 1990) was developed to provide a means of quickly screening for this domain of school functioning. It is a teacher rating scale of academic productivity and accuracy in major subject areas, with norms based on a sample of children from central Massachusetts (DuPaul, Rapport, & Perriello, 1991).

Self-Report Behavior Rating Scales for Children

Achenbach and Edelbrock (1987) have developed a rating scale quite similar to the CBCL, which is completed by children ages 11–18 years (Youth Self-Report Form). Most items are similar to those on the parent and teacher forms of the CBCL, except that they are worded in the first person. A later revision of this scale (Cross-Informant Version; Achenbach, 1991) now permits direct comparisons of results among the parent, teacher, and youth self-report forms of this popular rating scale. Research suggests that while such self-reports of ADHD children and teens are more deviant than the self-reports of youths without ADHD, the self-reports of problems by the ADHD youth, whether by interview or the CBCL Self-Report Form, are often less severe than the reports provided by parents and teachers (Fischer et al., 1993; Loeber, Green, Lahey, & Stouthamer-Loeber, 1991). The DBDRS could be given to children to complete about themselves (or used as a basis for such an interview) as a means of simply gathering the children's own view of their Disruptive Behavior Disorders. However, norms are not available and so the clinical utility of such self-ratings for the purpose of clinical diagnosis remains uncertain.

The reports of children about internalizing symptoms, such as anxiety and depression, are more reliable and likely to be more valid than the reports of parents and teachers about these symptoms in their children (Achenbach et al., 1987; Hinshaw, Han, Erhardt, & Huber, 1992). For this reason, the self-reports of defiant children and youth should still be collected, as such reports may have more pertinence to the diagnosis of comorbid disorders of children than to their defiant behavior itself.

Adaptive Behavior Scales and Inventories

Research has begun to show that a major area of life functioning affected by defiance and ADHD is the realm of general adaptive behavior (Barkley, DuPaul, & McMurray, 1990; Patterson, 1982; Roizen et al., 1994). Adaptive behavior often refers to the child's development of skills and abilities that will assist them in becoming more independent, responsible, and self-caring individuals. This domain often includes (1) self-help skills, such as dressing, bathing, feeding, and toileting requirements, as well as telling and using time and understanding and using money; (2) interpersonal skills, such as sharing, cooperation, and trust; (3) motor skills, such as fine motor (zipping, buttoning, drawing, printing, use of scissors, etc.) and gross motor abilities (walking, hopping, negotiating stairs, bike riding, etc.); (4) communication skills; and (5) social responsibility, such as degree of freedom permitted within and outside the home, running errands, performing chores, and so forth. So substantial and prevalent is this area of impairment among children with ADHD that Roizen et al. (1994) have even argued that a significant discrepancy between IQ and adaptive behavior scores (expressed as standard scores) may be a hallmark of ADHD.

Several instruments are available for the assessment of this domain of functioning. The Vineland Adaptive Behavior Inventory (Sparrow et al., 1984) is probably the most commonly used measure for assessing adaptive functioning. It is an interview, however, and takes considerable time to administer. Where time is of the essence, I have been using the NABC (Adams, 1984) for assessing this domain because of its greater ease of administration. This can be included as part of the packet of rating scales sent to parents in advance of the child's appointment for more efficient use of clinical time. The CBCL completed by parents (see above) also contains several short scales that provide a cursory screening of several areas of adaptive functioning (Activities, Social, and School) in children but is no substitute for the more in-depth coverage provided by the Vineland or NABC.

Peer Relationship Measures

As noted earlier, children with ODD, especially with comorbid ADHD, often demonstrate significant difficulties in their interactions with peers, and such difficulties are associated with an increased likelihood of persistence of their disorder (Biederman et al., 1996). A number of different methods for assessing peer relations have been employed in research with behavior problem children, such as direct observation and recording of social interactions, peer- and subject-completed sociometric ratings, and parent and teacher rating scales of children's social behavior. Most of these assessment methods have no norms and so would not be appropriate for use in the clinical evaluation of children with ADHD. Reviews of the methods for obtaining peer sociometric ratings can be found elsewhere (Asher & Coie, 1990; Newcomb, Bukowski, & Pattee, 1993). For clinical purposes, rating scales may offer the most convenient and cost-effective means for evaluating this important domain of childhood functioning. The CBCL and BASC rating forms described earlier contain scales that evaluate children's social behavior. As discussed above, norms are available for these scales, permitting their use in clinical settings. Three other scales that focus specifically on social skills are the Matson Evaluation of Social Skills with Youngsters (MESSY; Matson, Rotatori, & Helsel, 1983), the Taxonomy of Problem Social Situations for Children (TOPS; Dodge, McClaskey, & Feldman, 1985), and the Social Skills Rating System (Gresham & Elliott, 1990). The latter also has norms and a software scoring system, making it useful in clinical contexts.

Parent Self-Report Measures

It has become increasingly apparent that child behavioral disorders, their level of severity, and their response to interventions are, in part, a function of factors affecting parents and the family at large. As noted in the Introduction and particularly in Chapter 1, several types of psychiatric disorders are likely to occur more often among family members of a child with defiant behavior or ODD than in matched groups of control children. That these problems might further influence the frequency and severity of behavioral problems in defiant children has been demonstrated in numerous studies over the past 20 years. As discussed in Chapter 1, the extent of social isolation in mothers of behaviorally disturbed children influences the severity of the children's behavioral disorders as well as the outcomes of parent training. Others have also shown parental psychopathology and marital discord separately and interactively contribute to the decision to refer children for clinical assistance, the degree of conflict in parent–child interactions, and child antisocial behavior (see Chapter 1, Figure 1.4). The degree of resistance of parents to parent training is also dependent on such factors. Assessing the psychological integrity of parents, therefore, is an essential part of the clinical evaluation of defiant children, the differential diagnosis of their prevailing disorders, and the planning of treatments stemming from such assessments. Thus, the evaluation of children for defiant behavior is often a family assessment rather than one of the child alone. Although space does not permit a thorough discussion of the clinical assessment of adults and their disorders, brief mention will be made of some assessment methods that clinicians have found useful in providing at least a preliminary screening for certain important variables in the treatment of defiant children.

The instruments that assess the parents' own adjustment, discussed below, are completed by parents in my waiting room during the time their child is being interviewed. They are not mailed out in advance with the other rating scales, as the clinician will need to introduce the purpose of these self-report scales briefly to the parents so as not to offend them with the request for such sensitive information. Typically, I indicate to parents that having a complete understanding of a child's behavior problems requires learning more about both the children and their parents. This includes gaining more information about the parents' own psychological adjustment and how they view themselves in their role as parents. The rating scales below are then introduced as one means of gaining such information. Few parents refuse to complete these scales after an introduction of this type. To save time, some professionals prefer to send these self-report scales out to parents in advance of their appointment, at the same time as the child behavior questionnaires. If so, be sure to prepare a cover letter that sensitively explains to parents the need for obtaining such information about the parent. For instance, this letter might include the following statement:

"When completing the questionnaires pertaining to yourself and to other aspects of your marriage and family, please keep in mind that we are not trying to evaluate you. Instead, we are trying to learn as much as we can about the home environment in which your child lives. That home environment is very important in helping to understand the nature of the problems a child may be experiencing. Having such information allows us to make careful and well-informed recommendations about how best to help your child become more successful and better adjusted both at home and at school."

Parental ADHD and ODD

Family studies of the aggregation of psychiatric disorders among the biological relatives of children with ADHD and ODD have clearly demonstrated an increased prevalence of ADHD and ODD among the parents of these children (Biederman, Faraone, Keenan, & Tsuang, 1991; Faraone et al., 1993). In general, there seems to be at least a 40–50% chance that one of the two parents of the defiant child with ADHD will also have adult ADHD (15–20% of mothers and 25–30% of fathers). The manner in which ADHD in a parent might influence the behavior of an ADHD child specifically and the family environment more generally has not been well studied. Adults with ADHD have been shown to be more likely to have problems with anxiety, depression, personality disorders, alcohol use and abuse, and marital difficulties; to change their employment and residence more often; and to have less education and lower socioeconomic status than adults without ADHD (Barkley, Murphy, & Kwasnik, 1996; Murphy & Barkley, 1996a; Shekim, Asarnow, Hess, Zaucha, & Wheeler, 1990). Greater diversity and severity of psychopathology among parents is particularly apparent among the subgroup of ADHD children with comorbid ODD or

CD (Barkley, Anastopoulos, et al., 1992; Lahey et al., 1988). More severe ADHD seems to also be associated with younger age of parents (Murphy & Barkley, 1996b), suggesting that pregnancy during their own teenage or young adult years is more characteristic of parents of ADHD than non-ADHD children. It is not difficult to see that these factors, as well as the primary symptoms of ADHD, could influence the manner in which child behavior is managed within the family and the quality of home life for such children more generally. Ongoing research in our clinic suggests that where the parent has ADHD, the probability that the child with ADHD will also have ODD increases markedly. A recent clinical case (Evans et al., 1994) suggests that ADHD in a parent may interfere with the ability of that parent to benefit from a typical behavioral parent training program. Treatment of the parent's ADHD (with medication) resulted in greater success in subsequent retraining of the parent. These preliminary findings are suggestive of the importance of determining the presence of ADHD and even ODD in the parents of children undergoing evaluation for these disorders.

Recently, the DSM-IV symptom list for ADHD and ODD has been cast in the form of a behavior rating scale, and some limited regional norms on 720 adults, ages 17–84 years, have been collected (Murphy & Barkley, 1996c). This rating scale for adults, entitled the Adult Behavior Rating Scale, is provided in Part III. Adults complete the rating scale twice; once for their current behavioral adjustment and a second time for their recall of their childhood behavior between ages 5–12 years. Norms for current scores are provided in Table 2.2 and those for childhood recall scores are shown in Table 2.3. To score the scales, simply sum the number of points circled on the scale for each item across the items and check the tables for the threshold representing the 1.5 SDs above the mean for adults on each version. The Inattention items are 1–9, the Hyperactive–Impulsive items are 10–18, and the ODD items are 19–26. Again, clinically significant scores on these scales do not, by themselves, ensure the diagnosis of ADHD or ODD in a parent but should raise suspicion in the clinician's mind about such a possibility. If so, consideration should be given to referral of the parent for further evaluation and, possibly, treatment of adult ADHD or ODD, if necessary.

The use of such scales in the screening of parents of defiant children would be a useful first step in determining if the parents had ADHD. If the child meets diagnostic criteria for ADHD and these screening scales for ADHD in the parents proved positive (clinically significant), then referral of the parents for a more thorough evaluation and differential diagnosis might be in order. At the very least, positive findings from the screening would suggest the need to take them into account in treatment planning and parent training.

Marital Discord

Many instruments exist for evaluating marital discord between parents. The one most often used in research on childhood disorders has been the Locke–Wallace Marital Adjustment Scale (Locke & Wallace, 1959). As noted in Chapter 1, marital discord, parental separa-

TABLE 2.2. Means, Standard Deviations (*SD*), and Deviance Thresholds (+1.5 *SD*) by Age Group for the ADHD Summation Scores for Current Adult Symptoms Collapsed across Gender

Age (years)	Mean	*SD*	+1.5 *SD* cutoff	*N*
		Inattention		
17–29	6.3	4.7	13.4	275
30–49	5.5	4.4	11.4	316
50+	4.5	3.3	9.5	90
		Hyperactive–Impulsive		
17–29	8.5	4.7	15.6	276
30–49	6.7	4.3	13.2	309
50+	5.1	3.2	9.9	93
		Total ADHD score		
17–29	14.7	8.7	27.8	266
30–49	12.0	7.8	23.7	299
50+	9.5	5.8	18.2	87
		ODD score		
17–29	6.1	4.7	13.2	271
30–49	4.4	3.9	10.3	308
50+	3.1	2.9	7.5	91

Note. Data were collected on 720 adults of ages 17–84 years who were volunteers from among adults entering one of two sites of the Department of Motor Vehicles for new application or for renewal of their driver's license. The sample comprised 60% males and 40% females. The mean age was 35 years (*SD* = 13.2; range = 17–84), mean education was 14.1 years (*SD* = 2.8; range = 7–24), and mean Hollingshead Index of Social Position (for occupation only) was 40.6 (*SD* = 25.8; range = 10–90). The ethnic breakdown by sex was as follows: for males, 86% white, 5% black, 5% Hispanic, 1% Asian, and 3% other; for females, 85% white, 7% black, 2% Hispanic, 2% Asian, and 2% other. From Murphy and Barkley (1996c). Copyright 1997 by Multi-Health Systems, Inc. Reprinted by permission.

tion, and parental divorce are more common in parents of defiant children (Patterson, 1982; Patterson et al., 1992). Parents with such marital difficulties may have children with more severe defiant and aggressive behavior and such parents may also be less successful in parent training programs (see Chapter 1). Screening parents for marital problems, therefore, provides important clinical information to therapists contemplating a parent training program for such parents. Clinicians are encouraged to incorporate a screening instrument for marital discord into their assessment battery.

Parental Depression and General Psychological Distress

Parents of defiant children are frequently more depressed than those of normal children and this may affect their responsiveness to behavioral parent training programs (Forehand

TABLE 2.3. Means, Standard Deviations (*SD*), and Deviance Thresholds (+1.5 *SD*) by Age Group and Gender for the ADHD Summation Scores for Retrospective Recall of Childhood Symptoms

	Males					Females			
Ages (years)	Mean	*SD*	+1.5 *SD*	*N*		Mean	*SD*	+1.5 *SD*	*N*
				Inattention					
17–29	11.1	6.0	20.1	175		8.2	5.9	17.1	99
30–49	8.9	5.6	17.3	182		7.2	6.1	16.4	133
50+	6.1	4.0	12.1	55		3.5	3.1	8.2	38
				Hyperactive–Impulsive					
17–29	10.7	6.0	19.7	174		9.0	6.0	18.0	100
30–49	8.4	5.6	16.8	181		6.0	5.1	13.7	135
50+	5.6	3.4	10.7	55		3.3	2.7	7.4	39
				Total ADHD score					
17–29	21.8	11.3	38.8	173		17.3	11.4	34.4	96
30–49	17.3	10.4	32.9	177		13.2	10.8	29.4	129
50+	11.6	6.2	20.9	54		6.3	4.5	13.1	37
				ODD score					
17–29	9.3	6.1	18.5	171		7.2	5.9	16.1	102
30–49	6.9	5.5	15.2	178		4.8	4.9	12.2	133
50+	3.9	3.6	9.3	54		2.4	3.1	7.1	39

Note. From Murphy and Barkley (1996c). Copyright 1997 by Multi-Health Systems, Inc. Reprinted by permission.

& McMahon, 1981). A scale often used to provide a quick assessment of parental depression is the Beck Depression Inventory (Beck, Steer, & Garbin, 1988). Greater levels of psychopathology generally and psychiatric disorders specifically also have been found in parents of children with ADHD, many of whom also have ADHD (Breen & Barkley, 1988; Lahey et al., 1988). One means of assessing this area of parental difficulties is through the use of the Symptom Checklist 90—Revised (SCL-90-R; Derogatis, 1986). This instrument not only has a scale assessing depression in adults but also scales measuring other dimensions of adult psychopathology and psychological distress. Whether clinicians use this or some other scale, the assessment of parental psychological distress generally and psychiatric disorders particularly makes sense in view of their likely impact on the course and the implementation of the child's treatments, typically delivered via the parents.

Parental Stress

Research over the past 15 years suggests that parents of behavior problem children, especially those children with comorbid ODD and ADHD, report more stress in their families and their parental role than those of normal or clinic-referred non-ADHD children (Anastopoulos, Guevremont, Shelton, & DuPaul, 1992; Breen & Barkley, 1988; Fischer,

1990; Mash & Johnston, 1990). One measure frequently used in such research to evaluate this construct has been the Parenting Stress Index (PSI; Abidin, 1986). The original PSI is a 150-item multiple choice questionnaire, which can be scored to yield six scores pertaining to child behavioral characteristics (e.g., distractibility, mood, etc.), eight scores pertaining to maternal characteristics (e.g., depression, sense of competence as a parent, etc.), and two scores pertaining to situational and life stress events. These scores can be summed to yield three domain or summary scores, these being Child Domain, Mother Domain, and Total Stress. A shorter version of this scale is available (Abidin, 1986) and clinicians are encouraged to utilize it in evaluating parents of defiant children.

Summary of Assessment Methods

It should be clear from the foregoing that the assessment of defiant children is a complex and serious endeavor requiring adequate time (approximately 3 hours), knowledge of the relevant research and clinical literature as well as differential diagnosis, skillful clinical judgment in sorting out the pertinent issues, and sufficient resources to obtain multiple types of information from multiple sources (parents, child, teacher) using a variety of assessment methods. Where time and resources permit, direct observations of defiant and ADHD behaviors in the classroom could also be made by school personnel. At the very least, telephone contact with a child's teacher should be made to follow up on his/her responses to the child behavior rating scales and to obtain greater detail about the classroom behavior problems of the defiant child. To this list of assessment methods would be added those others necessary to address the specific problems often occurring in conjunction with defiant behavior or ODD in children.

Treatment Implications

A multimethod assessment protocol for defiant behavior in children will certainly reveal a variety of areas of deficits, excesses, and impairments requiring clinical intervention, and perhaps even more detailed behavioral assessment than has been noted here. The subsequent treatments undoubtedly will be based on those deficit areas found to be the most salient, the most significant to the concerns of the referral agent (e.g., parent, physician, teacher, etc.), or having the greatest impact on present and later adjustment. Such treatment recommendations may range from simple parent counseling concerning the disorder, in those children found to have no impairments, to residential treatment for those ODD or CD children having severe, chronic, or even dangerous forms of conduct problems or depression. Between these extremes, treatment recommendations may focus on improving any comorbid ADHD through stimulant medication or classroom behavioral interventions and improving the oppositional behavior of the defiant child through parent training in effective child management procedures. Many defiant children have peer relationship problems that might benefit from individual or group social skills training, provided such training were to be implemented within the school or neighborhood settings in which such skills should be used. The evaluation will, in most cases, reveal the need for multiple interventions for the child, or even the other family members, to address fully the issues raised therein. Regardless of the treatments indicated from the initial evaluation, ongoing, periodic reassessment using many of the methods noted above will be necessary in documenting change (or the lack thereof) throughout treatment, maintenance of treatment gains over time after treatment termination, and generalization (or the lack of it) of treatment effects to other problematic behaviors and environments.

Legal and Ethical Issues

Apart from the legal and ethical issues involved in the general practice of providing mental health services to children, several such issues may be somewhat more likely to occur in the evaluation of defiant children. The first of these involves the issue of custody or guardianship of the child as it pertains to who can request the evaluation of the child who may have defiance or ODD. Children with ODD, ADHD, or CD are more likely than average to come from families where the parents have separated or divorced or where significant marital discord may exist between the biological parents. As a result, the clinician must take care at the point of contact between the family and the clinic or professional to determine who has legal custody of the child and particularly the right to request mental health services on behalf of the minor. It must also be determined in cases of joint custody, an increasingly common status in divorce/custody situations, whether the nonresident parent has the right to dispute the referral for the evaluation, to consent to the evaluation, to attend on the day of appointment, and/or to have access to the final report. This right to review or dispute mental health services may also extend to the provision of treatment for the defiant child. Failing to attend to these issues before the evaluation can lead to great contentiousness, frustration, and even legal action among the parties to the evaluation that could have been avoided had greater care been taken to iron out these issues beforehand. Although these issues apply to all evaluations of children, they may be more likely to arise in families seeking assistance for ADHD children.

A second issue that also arises in all evaluations but may be more likely in cases involving ADHD is the duty of the clinician to report to state agencies any disclosure of suspected physical or sexual abuse or neglect of the child during the evaluation. Clinicians should routinely forewarn parents of this duty to report where it applies in a particular state *before* starting the formal evaluation procedures. In view of the greater stress that defiant or ODD children appear to pose for their parents as well as the greater psychological distress their parents are likely to report, the risk for abuse of defiant children may be higher than average. The greater likelihood of parental ADHD or other psychiatric disorders may further contribute to this risk, resulting in a greater likelihood that evaluations of children with disruptive behavior disorders may involve suspicions of abuse. Understanding such legal duties as they apply in a given state or region and taking care to exercise them properly yet with sensitivity to the larger clinical issues likely to be involved are the responsibility of any clinician involved in providing mental health services to children.

Increasingly over the past decade, ADHD children have been gaining access to government entitlements, sometimes thought of as legal rights, that make it necessary for clinicians to be well informed about these legal issues if they are properly and correctly to advise the parents and school staff involved in each case. For instance, children with ADHD are now entitled to formal special educational services in the United States under the Other Health Impaired Category of the Individuals with Disabilities in Education Act (1974). This, of course, is provided that their ADHD is sufficiently serious to interfere significantly with school performance. This is becoming commonly known throughout the United States. Less commonly understood is that such children also have legal protections and entitlements under Section 504 of the Rehabilitation Act of 1973 or the more recent Americans With Disabilities Act (1990) as it applies to the provision of an appropriate education to disabled children (see DuPaul & Stoner, 1994, and Latham & Latham, 1992, for discussions of these entitlements). And should ADHD children have a sufficiently severe disorder and reside in a family of low economic means, they may also be eligible for financial assistance under the Social Security Act. Space precludes a more complete explication of these legal entitlements here. The reader is referred to the excellent text by attorneys Latham and Latham (1992) for a fuller account of these matters. Suffice it to say here that clinicians working with defiant children who may have ADHD need to familiarize themselves with these various rights and entitlements if they are to be effective advocates for the children they serve.

A final legal issue related to defiant or ODD children pertains to their legal accountability for their actions in view of the argument made elsewhere (Barkley, 1996, in press) that their comorbid ADHD, which is likely to be present in most defiant children, is a developmental disorder of self-control. Should defiant children with ADHD be held legally responsible for the damage they may cause to property, the injury they may inflict on others, or the crimes they may commit? In short, is ADHD an excuse to behave irresponsibly without being held accountable for the consequences of one's actions? The answer is unclear and deserving of the attention of sharper legal minds than my own. It has been my opinion, however, that ADHD provides an explanation for why certain impulsive acts may have been committed but does not sufficiently disturb mental faculties to serve as an excuse from legal accountability, as might occur under the insanity defense, for example. Nor should ADHD be permitted to serve as an extenuating factor in the determination of guilt or the sentencing of an individual involved in criminal activities, particularly those involving violent crime. This opinion is predicated on the fact that the vast majority of children with ADHD, even those with comorbid ODD, do not become involved in violent crime as they grow up. Moreover, studies attempting to predict criminal conduct within samples of ADHD children followed to adulthood have either not been able to find adequate predictors of such outcomes or have found them to be so weak as to account for a paltry amount of variance in such outcomes. And those variables that may make a significant contribution to the prediction of criminal or delinquent behavior more often involve measures of parental and family dysfunction as well as social disadvantage and much less so, if at all, measures of ADHD symptoms. Until this matter receives greater legal scrutiny, it seems wise to view ADHD as one of several explanations for impulsive conduct but neither a direct, primary, nor immediate cause of criminal conduct by which the individual should be held unaccountable.

Screening Families for Parent Training

No single treatment program is successful for all clients. Recognizing this, researchers have studied those factors predicting success or failure within a parent training program such as this, as discussed in the Introduction. It should be obvious that conditions that affect the parents undergoing training will have some affect on their success in this program. For instance, parental psychiatric problems can interfere with that parent's ability to acquire and utilize the information in the training program, if not with attendance at the meetings themselves. Parents who are depressed, actively psychotic, or drug dependent during training will have a difficult time consistently utilizing the procedures with a behavior problem child, assuming they can follow them at all. Similarly, chronic health problems that affect their behavior may interfere to some degree with effective child management. Although there is little research on this issue, my clinical experience suggests that certain chronic medical conditions such as migraine headaches, epilepsy, premenstrual tension syndrome, and diabetes impair the implementation of the child management procedures. Several parental characteristics that have been repeatedly shown to predict poor outcome in training are depression, marital discord, maternal isolation (insularity) from the social community, and family socioeconomic status (Dumas & Wahler, 1983; Firestone & Witt, 1982; Forehand & McMahon, 1981; Strain et al., 1981). These variables relate to outcome in a linear way such that the greater their degree or severity within a family, the poorer the prognosis in training. Exercising careful judgment, the clinician must, when these factors are present, decide whether or not they should be addressed first (where possible), before beginning training.

In a similar way, certain conditions affecting the child may also impede the successful implementation of child management programs. Obviously, the type and severity of the child's behavior problems should be considered in the decision to undertake this or similar training regimens. If physical aggression and assault are sufficiently likely with a child, residential treatment would be a more prudent alternative to parent training, at least initially. Once the child's coercive behaviors have been brought under control within a more closely supervised environment, parent training could then serve as a therapy program for the transition of the child back into the home and the preparation of the parents for such a successful transition. Children with severe language delays or those with significant mental delays may not respond as well to this program because of its emphasis on compliance with verbal commands and rules. In my experience, children having a mental or language age of at least 2 years can respond successfully to these procedures. Greater time may be needed in working with the parents of such a child, particularly with practice sessions in the clinic, but improvement in child behavior in such cases is certainly possible.

Feasibility of Homework Assignments and Training Methods

Because the present program contains a variety of homework assignments to be done by parents, you must consider how feasible such assignments are for a given family and whether they should be modified to fit the individual characteristics of the parent or child. Less educated or intelligent parents may require less reading material but greater modeling and explanation of the procedures to understand them successfully. Parents with sensory or other handicaps may need special devices for recording their assignments, as in the case of using a tape recorder for recording the homework in situations where a parent is partially blind or illiterate.

How the methods are taught may also be slightly modified to fit the unique aspects of one's clinical situation or the family in training. A few parents may even need or wish to record the training sessions in order to review them between sessions. Both research (Webster-Stratton, 1984) and clinical experience suggest that in some instances videotaped instruction or examples of child management procedures can also be effective in parent training programs and is more cost effective than individual training of families. In general, you need to be sensitive to the individual and unique characteristics of each family and adjust the homework and training methods accordingly.

In so doing, you must decide whether individual or group parent training is to be used. Training individual families in these procedures is certainly effective, especially when augmented with live demonstrations of the methods and the opportunity for parents to practice these procedures with their child under the supervision of the therapist. Using a "Bug in the Ear" transmitting device combined with a clinic playroom, one-way mirror, and adjacent observation room greatly enhances the ability immediately to direct, shape, and reinforce parent management of children (Eyberg & Matarazzo, 1980).

However, the heavy caseloads of many clinicians do not always permit the training of individual families in all instances. As a result, group training may be necessary where four to eight sets of parents attend classes without their children. Group training has the advantage of being far more cost effective than individual training. It also allows parents an opportunity to commiserate about their experiences with the behavior problem children as well as to share possible solutions each has found in dealing with certain problems. Parents also develop a sense of camaraderie with others in the group that, in many cases, increases their motivation to carry out the homework assignments, particularly when they must describe their success at implementing the methods at the next group meeting. Studies comparing group versus individual training (Christensen, Johnson, Phillips, & Glasgow, 1980) have found the group training to be as effective while substantially reducing professional time involved in training. However, some parents may be easily intimidated by the more outspoken or successful couples in a group, or require more individualized in-struction in order to grasp the methods properly. Clinical experience with the program shows that not all families respond well to group training, and so some screening criteria for assigning parents to individual or group treatment should be exercised by the thera-pist. Generally, parents with more severely disturbed children, those of low educational or economic attainment, or those with multiple risk factors should be assigned at least ini-tially to individualized training programs.

Summary

This chapter has reviewed procedures for the assessment of defiant or ODD children. An approach is recommended that incorporates a structured interview, the use of rating scales to assess child deviance, and parent self-report measures of their own psychologi-cal adjustment. Some of these measures can be taken both prior to and after completion of the parent training program to evaluate improvements in parent–child relations. The assessment will also reveal several characteristics of the parents and children that should be considered for screening parents out of this child management training program because of their association with poorer outcomes in training. Other parent characteris-tics will have some bearing on how the homework assignments are individualized to that family's circumstances.

CHAPTER 3

Practical Considerations in Parent Training

Logistical and Practical Considerations in Training

Upon first learning this program, clinicians often ask several questions of practical import, such as whether it is necessary for both parents to attend the training sessions, if the sessions should be conducted in the clinic or the home, and how they should handle parents who fail to comply with the homework assignments. The answers to such questions clearly depend on many of the characteristics of a given family. However, some general advice can be offered.

Father Involvement in Training

Although I have found it useful for both parents to attend the training sessions where possible and appointments are provided late in the afternoon or early evening at times to accommodate working parents, research suggests it is not imperative in order for successful intervention to occur (Adesso & Lipson, 1981; Firestone, Kelly, & Fike, 1980; Martin, 1977). A review of the literature on father involvement in parent training (Horton, 1984) suggests that fathers are able to benefit from such training but show somewhat different patterns of behavioral change than are seen in mothers. Even if fathers do not attend, so long as mothers instruct the fathers in what they have learned in parent training classes, the child management behaviors of fathers can be improved. What appears to be crucial is whether the parent not attending, usually the father, is supportive of the attendance of the spouse and the implementation of the practices in the home (Horton, 1984). For now, it seems best to encourage fathers to attend the parent training sessions but treatment should not be denied to a mother merely because a father cannot attend.

In the case of single parents, this is not an issue. However, here the therapist may find that the single parent reports greater distress over the child's misbehavior, perhaps due to being unable to share such a burden with a supportive spouse. Supervision or training of the child may be impossible in the afternoon hours on weekdays should this parent also work outside the home, leaving the care of the child to sitters less skilled in child management tactics. Hence, success of the program may be somewhat diminished in some of these cases. Nevertheless, many single parents can and often do succeed in acquiring and effectively using the skills of this program with a defiant child.

Training in the Clinic or at Home?

Few studies have examined the issue of whether training in the clinic is as effective as that done in the family's home. What little research exists suggests that in-home training does not appreciably increase the effectiveness of parent training programs (Worland, Carney, Milich, & Grame, 1980), whereas it certainly increases the cost of the services. Increasingly in states, insurance companies and especially managed care plans are not likely to reimburse therapists for such out-of-office services, making the issue moot for those who derive their livelihood from such sources of compensation. My experience suggests that training in the clinic setting can be quite successful, less time consuming, less costly, and as effective as in-home training for most families. It has been my impression that going into the family's home may so artificially alter that environment that it differs little from the artificial surroundings of the clinic playroom in terms of enhancing treatment. Although an appreciation for the physical layout of the home and its condition can aid somewhat in individualizing certain management methods to that particular family, this benefit is often outweighed by the additional time and expense involved in going to the home. At this time, it appears that such in-home training should be reserved for the most severely behaviorally disruptive children, whose parents require such intensive efforts.

Group or Individual Family Training?

The increasingly cost-conscious nature in which mental health services are being provided to families demands that clinicians employ the most cost-effective means for conducting their treatment programs. If parent training programs can be offered in groups with equal efficacy, then this would be the preferred mode of service delivery for most families, given that more families can be treated for less time and expense in such a format. Fortunately, what evidence exists suggests that most families benefit equally as well from group training as from individual family parent training (Adesso & Lipson, 1981; Christensen et al., 1980; Cunningham, Bremner, & Boyle, 1995; Webster-Stratton, 1984). However, one study did not find group training to be as effective as individual parent training (Eyberg & Matarazzo, 1980) and found parents in such groups to be less satisfied than in individual family training. Yet several other studies have found no differences in consumer satisfaction ratings between individually trained and group trained parents (Webster-Stratton, 1984; Webster-Stratton, Kolpacoff, & Hollinsworth, 1985). Moreover, therapist time and expense for group training appears to be five to six times as cost effective as individual parent training programs conducted for the same number of families (Cunningham et al., 1995; Webster-Stratton, 1984), making a compelling case for group parent training as the first and primary mode of treatment delivery unless otherwise contraindicated. The use of videotaped models of child management skills as part of the group discussion in such training groups may enhance treatment effects beyond those achieved solely with group discussion of methods (Webster-Stratton et al., 1995). Also, the provision of such parent training classes in community settings (schools and community centers) versus hospitals or clinics may significantly increase the participation of minority and immigrant families, as well as that of families having more severe behavior problems with their children (Cunningham et al., 1995).

Managing Parental Noncompliance

The management of parental noncompliance with the treatment methods is not so easily addressed. When parents return to the next session of training without doing homework, how should the therapist handle the matter? In training more than 6,000 clinicians in this program over the past 20 years, the following methods have been offered and found useful. First, it should be clear that training in additional methods will not occur until the issue of noncompliance and its causes are addressed. In other words, parents are not permitted to advance to the next step in the program until they have mastered the step under discussion to the satisfaction of the clinician. Thus, it may take some families several weeks longer than others to advance through the steps of the program. For families in a group training program, one missed homework assignment or appointment is permitted. This family must meet with the therapist for an individual appointment to make up the missed appointment or homework assignment before the next group meeting. Families that miss more than one group meeting or homework assignment are then discontinued from the group and offered individual training if they so desire.

Second, the therapist needs to address within that individual session the reasons for failing to carry out the assignments. Often, legitimate reasons exist. In these instances, the session is a brief one and parents should be requested to try the assignment again in the coming week. Where little apparent reason exists for the parental noncompliance, the therapist may have to inquire skillfully about parental motivation for training or family stress events that may be interfering with training (such as marital discord, alcohol abuse, financial hardships, etc.). In some cases, training may be temporarily discontinued while the family stress event is managed or the parent is provided with a different intervention aimed at the stressor (e.g., maternal depression, marital discord, etc.).

A third method for coping with parental noncompliance is to establish a "breakage" fee (Patterson, 1982) whereby parents leave a fixed sum of money with the therapist and a portion of this is mailed to the parents' most-hated political or other organization for each missed assignment. Having the therapist keep the money may not be successful, because some parents feel that the therapist may deserve it for having been inconvenienced. This money is not part of the fee for therapy but is specifically identified for this purpose of motivating compliance. It is also possible to return a portion of the money to the parents for each assignment done correctly as a method of reinforcing parental compliance with the program. Some therapists may choose to implement both procedures with a given family, especially where parental motivation to participate in therapy is less than typical (e.g., court-ordered training or that imposed by a state social service agency).

In some cases where chronic parental noncompliance has occurred, this should be well documented and therapy discontinued. The parents may be told that, should they change their minds and decide to cooperate with training, they may return. Therapeutic services are far too expensive and their availability limited for the number of families in need of them to persist in nearly endless therapy sessions with uncooperative families.

Clinical and Stylistic Considerations

It is well known that treatment efforts can succeed or fail merely on the basis of the manner or style in which they are presented to a family. In fact, one major source of parental resistance to parent training programs has been shown to be therapist characteristics. Therapists who focus more on teaching and confronting parents during training may increase parental resistance to and noncompliance with training, as opposed to therapists who are more facilitative and supportive during the training program (Patterson & Forgatch, 1985). Research on this issue at the Oregon Social Learning Center by Patterson and colleagues suggests that parent trainers must engage in a delicate balancing act, "seeking an optimal level of teaching and confronting for individual parents and couples. That level would be just enough, but not too many, directives and confrontations to move the parents to change their family management practices" while still being facilitating and supportive enough to lower parental resistance and noncompliance (Patterson & Chamberlain, 1992, p. 31). Parents also appear to be more likely to drop out of training if assigned to therapist-trainees as opposed to experienced therapists (Frankel & Simmons, 1992).

Certainly, a large part of treatment efficacy can be traced to "placebo" or nonspecific factors associated with clinicians, their characteristics and manner of interacting with others, and the confidence and enthusiasm they project in their methods as they teach them. The specific treatment procedures, while obviously important, are of little effectiveness if clinicians cannot convincingly persuade parents of the importance of the procedures and their efficacy. These remarks and those that follow may seem obvious to skilled clinicians, but they are rarely stated in scientific papers on these treatment programs and may be overlooked by even the experienced clinician. Granted, there are varying preferences among clinicians on these issues of style. The points presented here are obviously ones that I favor and have found to work well in previous treatment cases. They should be viewed, therefore, as the suggestions they are, rather than as an inflexible set of rules to be applied equally to all cases.

I have found a general Socratic style of conveying concepts and behavioral principles to parents to be most helpful. This seems to help parents consider themselves an important part of the process of engineering programs for their children instead of feeling like fools or simpletons who must receive direct lecturing. Clinicians using such a Socratic style question the parents and lead them to the correct conclusion, concept, or method in such a manner that the parents feel that they have either achieved the solution on their own, or at least contributed to its discovery. It is felt that this method leaves a more lasting impression of the material with the parents and perhaps helps to maintain their motivation in treatment. Moreover, it avoids the implication of more directive styles of teaching that the parents are completely ignorant of child management principles—a myth that will be quickly dispelled by only a few cases of parent training. Although parents may not be able to use professional terminology to describe these principles, they are often accurate in describing the actual processes involved. Certainly, there will be times where a more directive style is necessary, particularly in describing and modeling a specific method or in outlining the homework assignment for a particular step of the program. When pressed for time, the therapist may elect to engage in direct lecturing in order to cover large amounts of material, but, in my experience, this is generally detrimental to parents' long-term acquisition of that material.

A corollary of this Socratic style is that professional jargon is to be avoided where possible. Efforts to teach parents the terminology of behavioral psychology hardly guarantee that they have understood the underlying principles sufficiently to ensure their use of them outside of therapy. Employing such jargon as "contingencies of reinforcement," "extinction," and "stimulus control" is overly pedantic and self-aggrandizing, and unnecessarily restricts the educational or intellectual range of parents to whom these methods can be taught. They are also likely to be viewed as dry, boring, or unintelligible by most parents who lack some college education, and this probably affects the compliance of these parents to therapy. There is also no empirical evidence to show that using such jargon enhances treatment efficacy. In the absence of such data, I feel that behavioral jargon is more of a hindrance than a help to teaching effective child management. It is left to you to decide whether, as a parent, you would prefer to hear that you should "periodically praise a child for complying with requests" or should "provide social secondary reinforcers on an intermittent schedule contingent upon the occurrence of compliant responses to verbal mands."

A Socratic method of teaching parents also seems to avoid a problem that is probably quite common in therapy—parental dependence on the therapist. When you alone design behavioral programs and then hand them to parents for use, the parents may fail to gain the problem-solving skills needed for dealing with present and future child behavior problems not immediately targeted in training. Week after week, such parents come to therapy to lay additional problems at the feet of the "great behavioral engineer" (you!), without ever understanding the basic principles used by you to design these programs. Such dependence will be hard to discontinue as treatment termination nears. Although this problem has not been widely studied, many clinicians would agree that parents who understand the principles and concepts that serve as the basis for a management method are more likely to use it than those who have been shown only the method.

Many behavioral therapists have noted that the principles they are attempting to convey to parents for use with their children are quite similar to those that they use in training the parents themselves. This obviously means that ample praise and appreciation (facilitation and support) are shown to parents upon their participation in therapeutic discussions, accomplishment of behavioral record keeping, and implementation of suggested treatment methods. Disapproval, confrontation, and even the withdrawal of reinforcers (such as breakage fees) are often contingent upon parental noncompliance with the suggested methods but must be, as noted earlier, delicately balanced with support and facilitation.

During each session, it is imperative that you periodically stop the discussion of new material and pause to assess the parents' understanding of what has been presented. In addition, you should invite the parents' opinions as to how they believe the method under discussion will fit into their particular schedule or style and how it may be used with their children in particular. This often reveals factors that would have hampered or precluded compliance to the method and suggests that the method may have to be modified to form a "best fit" with a particular family. The greater the discrepancy between the treatment demands and family lifestyles, the less compliance with treatment there will be. Although this may be obvious to the sophisticated reader, it is often overlooked in clinic situations when time is at a premium and caseloads are large.

A similar caution applies to leaping into new material at the beginning of a therapy session without first reviewing what has transpired in the life of a family since the last session or determining how well the homework assignment has succeeded. Overlooking such obvious stylistic precautions will often result in the errors being forcefully brought to your attention later in the session via a variety of client reactions, including resistance and further noncompliance. One such reaction may be apparent boredom or inattention to what clinicians are saying because of preoccupation with the as yet unacknowledged problem. Other clients may more assertively interrupt to present the complication, such as the fact that a spouse has deserted the home, a serious medical problem has arisen in a family member, or the method assigned for homework has resulted in serious misfortune for a parent or child. Such revelations often dictate that the course of therapy be altered or temporarily postponed until these new issues are addressed.

In discussing the behavioral methods, you should take care to invite the parents to modify or embellish them to meet specific needs in their family situation. Here it may be your turn to learn a thing or two from the clearly greater experience parents have with their particular children. This is nicely illustrated by a case in which parents were being taught to use a time out procedure in public settings, such as stores, where a chair or corner was not available for isolating the child contingent upon misbehavior. In this case, I explained that using a small pocket notebook to record the child's misbehavior and making the child aware of this beforehand might help. For every entry in the book, the child would have to spend 10 minutes in a time out chair upon his/her return home. In the next session, the parents explained that they had tried this method but added quite a novel twist to it. They had taken a Polaroid picture of their son seated in his time out chair at home and placed this in the spiral pocket notebook they were taking to the store. Before entering the store, they handed him the picture and reminded him that this was where he would wind up at home if misbehavior occurred. I have found this embellishment to be of such practical value that it is now described to each new set of parents trained in this approach as part of the handout for the session on public misbehavior (Step 7. Anticipating Problems: Managing Children in Public Places). As noted earlier, parents are rarely ignorant of effective behavioral methods or principles and can serve as satisfactory "cotherapists" at some points in therapy. I have found it useful to explain the need for such collaboration at the beginning of therapy. This serves a secondary function of letting parents know that clinicians do not necessarily have all of the answers to their children's problems. Although the clinician may be an expert about general behavioral principles and technology, the parents are the obvious experts about their particular children, their habits, their temperaments, and their reaction patterns. Acting as if parents know nothing about child behavior principles is both patronizing and professionally naive. Without the integration of information from both sets of "experts," therapy is much less likely to succeed.

It almost goes without saying that interspersed throughout therapy should be periodic expressions of empathy for parents' or families' current circumstances, and especially for the work needed to use this program well. Acknowledgements that the methods being discussed are easy to read but not so easy to put into effect are helpful. Reminders about the importance of doing homework regularly and practicing the methods should also be periodically given. Often it can be helpful to draw analogies between learning child management skills and acquiring new skills with musical instruments or recreational sports. Parents are usually quick to give therapists total credit for any success at improving their children's behavior. It should be made obvious to them that the success is partly if not solely due to their use of the behavioral method, because no tool left on the shelf miraculously fixes a problem. In short, then, therapist facilitative and supportive behaviors are an important part of enhancing parent participation in and compliance with the parent training program.

Scheduling Sessions

Although parent training sessions may be scheduled throughout your typical clinic day, I have found it useful to set aside late afternoon times for this program so as to encourage fathers to attend without jeopardizing their employment, and mothers as well, should they also be employed outside the home. Training of individual families is done through weekly visits typically lasting 1 hour. Parent training groups should be the preferred mode of treatment, however. Such groups should have weekly meetings lasting 2–2.5 hours. Although research has shown such groups to be effective with up to 18 families per group when offered in community settings (Cunningham et al., 1995), in clinical settings such as mine the preferred group size is no more than 6–10 families.

The decision to place a family in group versus individual therapy often revolves around issues of parental educational level; type, number, and severity of the child's problems; degree of family stress; and the extent of individual attention a family may require. For cost-effective reasons, it may be wisest to enroll most or all families in group parent training first and then consider retraining any nonresponders using a more individualized delivery.

Summary

In this chapter, I have reviewed various practical issues involved in the clinical implementation of the program, such as the setting and format in which training is provided, ways to cope with parental noncompliance, stylistic considerations in training, and the scheduling of therapy sessions. I emphasize a sensible, pragmatic, and unpretentious approach to teaching that makes clear to parents the demands of the program and the specific methods to use, while remaining empathic and facilitative of parental participation.

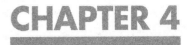

CHAPTER 4

An Overview of the Parent Training Program

Before reviewing in detail the specific methods to be taught in each step of the program, it is necessary to examine the basic concepts upon which the training program is built, the rationale for the sequence of the steps, and the schedule of activities occurring within each session.

Concepts Underlying Child Management Training

Several important principles of child management are interwoven throughout the training sequence. To grasp fully the program's orientation and potential power, practitioners should know these concepts in advance.

Make Consequences Immediate

Consequences for child behavior, be they positive or negative, must be provided immediately if parents are to gain effective control over inappropriate behavior. You should repeatedly stress that parents need to provide consequences for a child immediately after the occurrence of the targeted behavior, rather than waiting until several minutes or hours later to confront the problem or reward the appropriate behavior. Because of the hectic lifestyles of many families, most parents delay dealing with behaviors, especially positive or appropriate ones. They are often much quicker to attend to undesirable or especially intrusive behaviors. But, even with these, they often wait until after the fourth or fifth repetition of a command before providing consequences for their children's noncompliance. In short, the more quickly a parent can provide consequences to a child, the greater the control they will exert over that child's behavior.

Make Consequences Specific

Parents are also instructed that consequences, especially verbal or social ones, should be quite specific. Both praise and criticism should refer to the behavior at issue, instead of being vague, general, or nebulous references to the children themselves, their general behavior, or their personal integrity. Similarly, with punishment, the consequences should be tailored to fit the transgression and not be based on the parents' level of impatience or frustration over this or prior episodes of misbehavior.

Make Consequences Consistent

Virtually all behavioral approaches to parent training stress the concept of consistency of consequences as a key to greater control of child behavior. This refers to consistency across settings, over time, and between parents. Consistency across settings simply means that if a behavior occurs that is generally punished in one environment, say the home, then it is also punished in other environments, such as stores. Although there may be occasional exceptions to this rule, it is generally a good policy for parents to respond to child behaviors similarly across various social contexts. This is often contrary to the practice of many parents who handle a problem one way while at home and a different way when in public places where others may observe them. Such a practice directly trains the child as to which situation will prove successful for the display of misbehavior.

Consistency over time simply refers to the fact that parental standards about acceptable and unacceptable behavior in children should not vary too greatly from one moment to the next. Although these standards will change as a function of developmental changes in the child, over more immediate time periods it is necessary for parents to provide consequences for behavior as consistently as possible. Child behavior that is defined as unacceptable on one day should not be arbitrarily tolerated or even reinforced on another. For instance, punishing a child for "raiding" the refrigerator because a parent has a headache, while ignoring or actually assisting a visit to the refrigerator at a future time is a ludicrous practice, which only greatly reinforces such rule violations in the home. The converse is also true in that a behavior that is rewarded today should be so in the future and should certainly not be subjected to punishment later.

Consistency between parents in the rules they establish for children and the consequences they employ for their adherence or violation is also important. Quite frequently, mothers tend to manage the problems they experience with a child in ways very different from those of the fathers; this often leads to conflicts not only in the development of a consistent set of rules for the children but also in the marital relationship.

Establish Incentive Programs before Punishment

Another concept is that punishment for inappropriate behavior should not be introduced in the home unless the parents have established a specific program for rewarding the appropriate alternative behavior. Most parents phrase their concerns about child behavior in the negative, specifying what it is they dislike about a child. This naturally leads to a consideration of punishment methods to suppress the unwanted behavior. As a result, punishment is the major type of interaction in the family and children rarely receive reinforcement for whatever acceptable behavior may be shown. Furthermore, punishment appears to lose its effectiveness in such circumstances where the family environment is devoid of positive incentives for appropriate conduct. By teaching parents to rephrase their complaints about child behavior into their prosocial or appropriate alternatives, the natural response is then one of thinking of incentives to encourage an increase in this behavior. Only then should consideration be given to punishment methods for reducing the unacceptable behavior by the child. This is especially true in those sessions where punishment is being taught, lest parents perceive the therapist as advocating the use of punishment as a primary response to misconduct by children.

Anticipate and Plan for Misbehavior

The experienced clinician recognizes that many parents are as impulsive in their reactions to child misbehavior as their children are in reacting to various events. This results in parents spending tremendous amounts of time in managing misbehavior while investing minimal, if any, time in analyzing, anticipating, and possibly preventing those situations in which the children are likely to create problems. If parents were to anticipate problematic encounters, they might develop methods that would reduce the probability of those problems developing. Perhaps this apparent lack of forethought or anticipation is merely the result of being so overwhelmed with incorrigible behavior that it is difficult to "take the offensive" and try to anticipate and ward off future problems in a particular setting. Or, perhaps, it results from some parents having forms of psychopathology similar to those of their children (i.e., ADHD and ODD), making the parent more impulsive and immature compared to other parents, just as the children are relative to their own peers. Regardless of the reasons, such lack of forethought contributes to many of the difficulties parents have in dealing with children in particular places, such as in stores, restaurants, and so forth. It is necessary periodically to discuss with parents this issue of thinking ahead about problem situations and preparing a plan of behavior management for the child before entering the potential problem situation. This is certainly contrary to the more typical situation of waiting until the disruptive or unmanageable behavior occurs and then trying to determine what to do about it; that strategy amounts to being "too little, too late" in dealing with defiant children.

Recognize That Family Interactions Are Reciprocal

Another concept conveyed to parents throughout the program is that of reciprocity of interactions within families. Parents often have a unilateral view of the causes of child behavior problems—either they caused the problem or it is all the child's fault. You must periodically emphasize that interaction patterns within families are quite complex and not especially well understood at this time. However, there are strong indications that parents' behavior toward a child is partly a function of that child's behavior toward them; the child's temperament, physical characteristics, and abilities; and prior experiences with that child (Bell & Harper, 1977; Patterson, 1982). Similarly, the child's behavior is partly a function of how the parent treats the child; the parent's own temperament, physical characteristics, and abilities; and prior experiences with that parent. Because of this bidirectional influence between parent and child, it is difficult to assign blame to either party for the current state of conflict. Hence, no time in this program is spent in blaming parents *or* children for interaction problems, a practice that is of no constructive worth in overcoming those problems. Instead, all parties to the problematic interaction bear some responsibility for its resolution. That parents are chosen as the major focus of change has more to do with convenience and their motivation to alter the problem interactions than it does with finding fault with their child management skills.

In summary, the following general concepts concerning child management deserve periodic emphasis throughout the course of therapy: (1) making consequences immediate and specific; (2) making consequences consistent across settings, over time, and between parents; (3) establishing incentive programs for appropriate behavior before implementing punishment methods to suppress its unacceptable alternative; (5) anticipating potential problem situations and preparing a plan of action ahead of time; and (6) emphasizing that interaction patterns in families are reciprocal systems, thus making fault finding with parents or children of little constructive value.

Sequence of Steps within the Program

There are 10 steps to the core parent training program. The program can be taught as one self-contained unit with therapy terminating after the final session, or it can be integrated into an ongoing family therapy or parent counseling program designed to address other difficulties in the family, marriage, or parent's own personal life. In some cases, it may be necessary to change to other forms of therapy after these steps are completed in order to address other problems of the child, such as enuresis or encopresis, noncompliance with medical treatments, or school performance issues. In any case, the sequence of the procedures within this core program should remain essentially the same. Much research and clinical experience have been invested in constructing the steps of the program and their sequence, and they are deliberately presented in this order for significant reasons. Although it is possible that some families may not require all steps of the program due to the mild nature of the child's noncompliance, the training chosen for any particular case should follow this order. The justification is that the initial sessions emphasize the development of positive behavior management methods within the family, especially the use of incentives for compliance with rules and commands, while later sessions deal specifically with punishment techniques. Inverting the sequence such that punishment is taught first may result in an excessive reliance by parents on punishment throughout the entire program and, perhaps, ultimately to a lessened effectiveness of such techniques. By establishing a home environment rich with incentives for appropriate behavior, the subsequent introduction of selective, mild punishment appears to go more smoothly and effectively.

In cases of only minor noncompliance by a child, a therapist may choose to train the parents only in the use of praise for acceptable compliance and appropriate child behavior and then skip to the use of the time out procedure for the occasional noncompliance by the child. In such instances, parents will generally find these two procedures to be sufficiently effective, and they will not need the more intense contingency management procedures and discussions of the causes of child misbehavior. Here, even the time out procedure need not be as dramatic or intense as it is in the usual approach because the minor level of non-compliance does not warrant such intensity. Occasionally, the therapist may wish to implement the home poker chip or point systems to augment the enhanced use of praise with these children, which is often very successful. Nonetheless, even in such mild cases, the sequence remains the same—positive reinforcement and incentive methods are taught first, before the punishment procedures are introduced.

In most cases, the complete sequence of steps should be taught, as follows:

- *Step 1: Why Children Misbehave.* This session is intended to teach parents the typical causes of child misbehavior, how these causes interact, and what parents can do to begin identifying such causes within their own children and families.

- *Step 2: Pay Attention!* The value of parental attention to the child is quite low at the beginning of therapy, making it almost useless in many cases as a way of motivating better child behavior. This session is intended to train parents in ways of eliminating ineffective or even detrimental attending while increasing more effective forms of attending to and appreciating child behavior.

- *Step 3: Increasing Compliance and Independent Play.* Once parents develop more valuable and effective attending skills, these skills are then directed specifically at improving child compliance by having parents contingently respond to it with acknowledgement, appreciation, and praise when it occurs. This step also provides parents with instruction in how to attend to children at those times when the children are *not* interrupting or bothering their parents while parents are engaged in an activity (e.g., talking on the telephone, working in the kitchen, speaking to a visitor, etc.). By interrupting their own activities frequently to attend positively to child independent play, parents are able to increase those periods of time when children are not bothersome during parental activities.

- *Step 4: When Praise Is Not Enough: Poker Chips and Points.* Recognizing that praise and attention are rarely sufficient by themselves to motivate better compliance in clinic-referred children, the therapist now requires the parents to implement a highly effective motivational program that enlists a variety of rewards and incentives readily available within the home to increase child compliance with commands, rules, chores, and codes of social conduct in the home. This program is quite useful for children of mental ages of 4 years and older. Poker chips are used as tokens for 4- to 8-year-olds while 9- to 11-year-olds are provided with "points" recorded in a notebook. Children earn points or chips contingent upon acceptable compliance with rules and commands and may use these tokens for the purchase of daily, weekly, or long-term privileges and rewards.

- *Step 5: Time Out and Other Disciplinary Methods.* In this step, parents receive instruction in how to use the token system described above as a form of punishment, or "response cost" (i.e., penalties in the token program are assessed for inappropriate behavior). However, much of this step is devoted to a detailed discussion of a procedure known as "time out from reinforcement," or simply "time out." This procedure involves immediately isolating the child to a chair in a dull corner of the home upon the occurrence of noncompliance or unacceptable social conduct. Parents may only use this time out method for one or two misbehaviors, utilizing fines within the token system for managing other types of misconduct for now.

- *Step 6: Extending Time Out to Other Misbehavior.* Once parents are effectively employing the time out technique, they are permitted to expand its use to an additional one or two misbehaviors by the children. Where problems have been encountered in using the method, much of this session is devoted to troubleshooting the problems with implementing time out and correcting them.

- *Step 7: Anticipating Problems: Managing Children in Public Places.* Up to this point, parents have been reminded to use the treatment procedures only within the home. At this step, parents are now trained to use slightly modified versions of the techniques for managing child misbehavior in public places, such as stores, restaurants, church, and so forth. The training incorporates a method known as "think aloud–think ahead" wherein parents establish a plan for themselves for managing misconduct immediately before entering any public building, share the plan with the children, and then adhere to their plan while in the public place. Included in this plan is often a set of positive or constructive activities (helping) given to the child so as to keep them busy during the upcoming situation. While parents are initially instructed in this procedure for use out of the home, they are also taught to use it within the home just before a major transition in household activities is expected to occur involving the child (e.g., visitors coming to the home, going from child play to school homework, extended chore performance, bathtime, bedtime, or other major activity shift).

- *Step 8: Improving School Performance from Home: The Daily School Behavior Report Card.* This session is optional and intended for school-age children where problem behaviors may be occurring at school. Although parents cannot always be expected to help teachers with the classroom management of their children, there is a way in which parents can utilize incentives within the home to reinforce better child behavior in the classroom. This is done through the use of a daily school behavior report card combined with a home-based reward program (typically, the token system noted above). This session is used to discuss the child's school behavior and teach parents to use a daily school report card with their home token system.

- *Step 9: Handling Future Behavior Problems.* Parents are now briefly instructed in how these procedures might be used for other behavior problems that the child does not now have. In addition, parents are quizzed as to how they might design a behavior change program based on the methods they have been using.

- *Step 10: Booster Session and Follow-Up Meetings.* Parents are requested to return for a 1-month booster session to assess their adherence to the treatment methods, plan on the fading out of the home token system should that be appropriate, and aid parents in troubleshooting any problems they may now be encountering. Parents are cautioned about slippage or regression in their management tactics—the return to previously ineffective and punishment dominated methods—and are encouraged to remain with the treatment techniques for as long as possible. They are then scheduled to be seen in 3 months for a follow-up visit in which progress and problems are reassessed (and retreated if necessary).

Sequence of Activities within Each Session

Other than the first step, the sessions follow a standard pattern of events. Whether group or individual family training is selected as the teaching format, each session begins with a review of the previous week's homework assignment and any other events the family may wish to share with you (or the group). Problems that may have arisen in implementing prior instructions are discussed and resolved. In individual family training, should parents fail to have done the homework, this issue is addressed, as discussed above, and the parents are reassigned this homework for the next week. When this occurs, no new material would be discussed in the session. In a group training format, the therapist would schedule a separate individual session with any family failing to do the homework so as to discuss this issue privately and determine whether this family should proceed further with training. That family remains in the group for this session, however. If homework was done satisfactorily, the new material, concepts, and methods are introduced, regardless of which teaching format is employed. Where appropriate, you should model or demonstrate these methods. Some therapists may choose to use videotaped demonstrations of the techniques to enhance the parents' acquisition of the method (see Webster-Stratton, 1984; Webster-Stratton et al., 1989).

If the training is being done with an individual family, then at this stage of the session some practice of the methods within the sessions is encouraged. The parent and child can go to a playroom and the parent would practice the methods with the child under your supervision, usually using a one-way mirror if available. Any of several transmitter devices may be used for this purpose. These usually involve a small transmitter and microphone installed in the observation room connected to an antennae in the adjacent playroom. The parent is given direct and immediate feedback during practice using a small hearing aid (receiver) worn by the parent, which receives voice transmissions from the adjoining observation room. Should this resource not be available, simply observing the parents and child in a portion of your office for 15 minutes and then discussing with the parent the impressions of the performance can serve the same purpose. You would then discuss any problems the parents might envision in implementing the technique in their home during the coming week. In a parent group, no practice need occur at this point. Instead, group discussion of the methods and any problems each family anticipates encountering when implementing this procedure at home would be the focal points of the group activity at this time.

Subsequently, the homework for the coming week is assigned and questions regarding it are resolved. Ample praise, encouragement, and positive feedback are provided throughout each session for the parents' participation in discussions, compliance with the instructions and homework, and general cooperation with the training program.

Summary

This chapter briefly describes the important concepts or principles upon which the treatment methods are founded, as well as the 10 steps of the program and their sequence. Emphasis is placed on adhering to the particular pattern of training, as it is important in its own right, beyond simply the methods being taught. Which methods are introduced in what sequence is often crucial to enhancing the effectiveness of the total program. A method for organizing the material to be taught within each step is also presented.

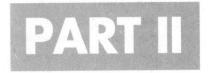

Guidelines for Therapists in Conducting The Program

This section provides detailed guidelines for conducting each of the steps of this parent training program. Within each step, goals of that step are specifically stated, an outline for use in the session is provided, and specific instructions for conducting that step are then described. You will want to review the sequence of activities within each session as described in Chapter 4 of Part I of this manual before beginning treatment with each new case. You will also find it helpful to refer to the outline provided for each step while conducting that step of the program so as to ensure that all of the important information is reviewed with the parents. Finally, the parent handouts that accompany each step are set forth in Part IV of this manual. These can be photocopied as needed for distribution to your clients as part of your treatment of them with this program.

Why Children Misbehave

Goals

1. To educate parents concerning the causes of children's defiant behavior.
2. To urge parents to identify those causes of or contributors to defiant behavior that may exist in their families.
3. To encourage parents to begin to remedy those causes of defiance that can be rectified within their families.

Materials Required

- Home Situations Questionnaire
- Disruptive Behavior Disorders Rating Scale—Parent Form
- Parent Handouts for Step 1
    Profile of Child and Parent Characteristics
    Family Problems Inventory
- Diagram of Oppositional Defiant Interaction

Step Outline

- Review events since the evaluation
- Brief reassessment of child disruptive behavior (rating scales)
- Open discussion of parents' views of the causes of misbehavior
- Presentation of a model for understanding child misbehavior
    The child's characteristics
    The parents' characteristics
    Situational consequences

Family stress events
The reciprocal interaction among these factors

- The goal of therapy: Designing a "best fit" between parent, child, and the family's circumstances

- Some handicaps are behavioral: The need for a prosthetic social environment when ADHD coexists with defiance

Homework

- Family Problems Inventory
- Childproofing the home

Review of Events Since the Evaluation

The beginning of each session is always an invitation to the parents to describe any significant events that have transpired since the parents last met with the therapist. In most cases, this will have been the time of the child's initial clinical evaluation. In some cases, the family will have been seeing the therapist regularly in ongoing treatment, the focus of which is now shifting to direct instruction in child management skills. Because each session begins with this review of prior events, it will receive no further discussion in the description of subsequent steps in the program.

Reassessment of Child Disruptive Behavior

So as to monitor the family's response to parent training, I advise clinicians to administer two rating scales of child behavior every three sessions, beginning in Session 1 (Sessions 1, 4, 7, and 10 and 1–month booster session). Two scales should be given, both of which are provided in Part III: (1) the DBDRS-PF and (2) the HSQ. These scales take very little time to complete but provide a brief reevaluation of the type, severity, and pervasiveness of the child's behavioral problems. This information helps to guide the therapist's discussions with the parents and also serves as a measure of therapy effectiveness with this family. Research shows that clinicians can expect a decline in the severity of ratings on the scales between their first use in the child's initial evaluation and their completion again at the start of training (Session 1). Such practice effects are commonplace and, if not detected in this way, are often misattributed to the results of therapy. By giving these two scales again before starting formal parent training, the second administration of these scales now becomes the baseline against which therapeutic effectiveness for a particular family can be more accurately measured in subsequent training sessions. So, photocopy five sets of these two scales to have on hand in the patient's files to be completed by parents periodically throughout training at the sessions noted above.

Open Discussion of Parents' Views of the Causes of Misbehavior

Although it will be a major goal of this session to provide parents with a framework in which to understand child misbehavior and psychopathology, it is useful to assess the parents' own perceptions of why children develop significant behavioral problems. Initially, you should invite parents to discuss openly what causes they believe lead to misbehavior in their children. These should be written down by the therapist so that they can be placed within the model of causes of misbehavior to be presented later. In my experience, parents are quick to identify "getting attention" as a major reason children display disruptive behavior. Although this is correct in some instances, you will later show how coercive interactions actually develop from escape/avoidance learning (negative reinforcement) in children rather than merely to get adult attention. Other parents will blame themselves, identifying "poor parenting" as a major cause of noncompliance. For now, simply note this comment but be sure to respond to it later after explaining the model of misbehavior below. At that point, you will want to disspell this notion somewhat by showing how complex the causes of misbehavior happen to be. A few parents will correctly note that some children seem destined to have behavioral difficulties from birth; inviting parents to elaborate on this theme is a helpful transition into your presentation of the model below.

A Model for Understanding Child Misbehavior

Although research in developmental psychopathology and disruptive child behavior (see Chapters 1 and 2) has identified myriad causes of child misbehavior, they can be grouped into four major factors to permit their ease of teaching to parents.

The Child's Psychological Characteristics

Some children are born with a certain predilection toward disruptive behavior specifically and psychopathology more generally. Such children may have inherited predispositions toward thought disorders, psychotic behavior, and intellectual delay, as well as attention deficits, impulsivity, and irritability to name but a few, given the evidence presently available on the familial nature of these disorders. Other children appear to manifest difficult temperaments that bring them into conflict with their caregivers very early in the their development. "Temperament" here refers to the children's activity level, general attention span, emotionality and irritability, sociability, response to stimulation, and habit regularity.

At this point, you should provide parents with the first handout for this step for them to follow in this discussion. (Parent handouts for all steps are to be found in Part IV. In addition the handouts have been translated into Spanish and are available as a supplement to this manual from the publisher. Note that this instruction will not be repeated in subsequent steps.) Be sure to explain that these aspects of temperament appear to be inborn characteristics of the children to a great extent, are often easily identifiable within the first 6 months of life, and are stable over many years. Each characteristic should be briefly explained. After each, have parents indicate on the handout whether that characteristic is a problem for their child. Parents can rate each feature on a scale of 1 (mild or no problem) to 10 (severe or very serious problem).

Among the many characteristics of children that may contribute toward a more stressful parent–child interaction, and so to a greater risk for conflict with others, are the obvious ones of a child's health or chronic medical problems, physical disabilities, developmental delays, and even difficulties with impulse control. Though obvious, all should be discussed briefly with the parents in taking stock of those characteristics that may be important in understanding any conflict the child has within the family or with others outside the home.

In the handout, "attention span" refers to the average duration of time a child usually spends watching, listening to, manipulating, or otherwise behaving toward stimuli in the environment. In particular, the child's persistence in attending to activities is important as an early marker of later self-control and ADHD, the latter often characterized as involving poor persistence of attention and distractibility. "Activity level" here refers to the specific level of motor activity shown by the child. "Social behavior problems" refer to the child's general level of interest in others as opposed to things. Eye contact with others, initiating interactions toward others, and generally viewing others as more important to interact with in a situation than are objects are all aspects of sociability in children. In particular, how responsive the child is to the social feedback he/she receive from others is an important part of this construct.

Emotional problems and irritability should be discussed with an emphasis on response to stimulation. The child's general reaction to noise; tactile, auditory, or visual stimulation; movement produced by others, and so forth, are all important factors. Some children withdraw when only lightly stimulated by their environment. They are quite sensorially defensive, "skittish," and oversensitive to environmental stimuli. Others may cry easily when stimulated or become irritable . Still others may seek out stimulation, explore novel aspects of an environment vigorously, and in some cases enjoy mild stimulation from others. The consistency of the child's biological habits, such as eating, sleeping, and elimination patterns, should be discussed to determine habit regularity. Some children are fussy or picky eaters, develop colic easily, have shorter-than-normal sleep patterns, or have irregular habits of elimination. Obviously, these can add additional stress to caregivers in trying to establish an infant or young child's "daily routine." Emotional problems and irritability also are clues to the child's general emotional reactions to events within the environment. How quickly or easily is this child moved to emotional displays? Some children are generally irritable, cry often, are hard to console when upset, and just generally emote very easily and often to excess.

Explain to parents that these are overlapping features of children and are simply lumped together into one general impression of a child's temperament (very easy to very difficult). The greater a child deviates from normal on these dimensions of temperament and the more dimensions on which he is deviant, the greater is the likelihood of conflict developing with the parents. Such parent–child conflicts will often be greatest for that parent who must make the most daily demands on the child. Such demands are more likely to elicit the child's negative temperament, resulting in that parent having a far more negative view of the child's manageability than the parent having fewer daily management encounters with the child. It is not hard to see how this could lead to marital strife, with one parent receiving the brunt of the child's negative temperament.

It is also not difficult to see how such child characteristics could lead to conflict with other adults and the community in which the child resides. In a society that values controlled, well-channeled activity levels; sustained attention; reasonably regulated emotional reactions; moderate degrees of sociability; curiosity in healthy but channeled ways; and predictable regularity of habits that lead to easy caretaking, an infant or child who is seriously deviant or negative in these areas is destined to have great difficulties in social and familial adjustment, no matter what the parents are like. In short, from birth onward, some children with negative temperaments have a high probability of encountering or contributing to conflict with their social environment. You are trying to determine through this survey if this might be such a child and to have the parents appreciate this likely possibility. In essence, this shows it is not entirely the parents' fault that conflict may have arisen with this child.

The *physical characteristics* of a child are another feature that may predispose children toward misbehavior. The child's physical appearance, motor coordination, strength, stamina, and general physical abilities are well-recognized factors in determining to some degree how others will react to him/her, at least initially. A child who is unattractive, uncoordinated, weak, or generally different from others in physical abilities will have fewer positive initial interactions with others, may accidentally damage property, may be unable to participate in children's play or games gracefully, and may be at risk for failure in certain academic areas (e.g., handwriting). Such problems not only result in initial negative feedback or dislike, or even rejection or outright hostility by others toward the child so afflicted, but can render damage to the child's self-esteem and his/her desire to be accepted by family, peers, and society. The mere fact that a child may resemble someone else in the family who was disliked (a former husband, for instance) may subtly affect the types and manner of interactions he/she may receive from other family members (the mother in this case).

Finally, a child's *developmental abilities* may place him/her at risk for behavioral problems. Like physical characteristics, developmental competencies also affect how others initially perceive the children and subsequently interact with them. For instance, a mild delay in language development or impaired speech expression, less than average intellect, or poor visual–motor coordination may result in poor social acceptance, teasing, or other forms of social maltreatment. Such delays may also affect a child's social problem-solving abilities, ability to understand and comply with parental commands and requests, or ability to learn appropriate habits or emotional control. These may lead directly to conflict with caregivers and others with whom the child interacts. Parents should be invited to give examples in each of these areas as to specific characteristics they may have noted that affect children's social behavior and acceptance.

At this point, ask the parents to describe their child briefly in each of these areas in order to see what factors the child may already have that could predispose him/her toward misconduct. Use the Profile of Child Characteristics provided with the printed handouts that accompany this manual for this purpose.

The Parents' Characteristics

You should now discuss with the parents the fact that their own characteristics play some role in the development or maintenance of behavior problems in their children. Following the same outline of characteristics used above in describing the behavior problem child, discuss how parents may themselves have certain inherited predispositions to personal psychological disorders, temperamental characteristics, physical features or disabilities, or developmental disabilities that place them at risk for contributing to behavioral difficulties in their children. These characteristics can have a detrimental effect on the parents' consistency and effectiveness in managing child misbehavior when it arises. Virtually the same difficulties that may plague the behavior problem child in these areas can also be seen in some parents.

Encourage parents to provide specific characteristics within these categories that they recognize may contribute to the problems parents have managing children, especially those with behavioral disorders. Then have the parents complete the Profile of Parent Characteristics that accompanies the handouts with this manual. The intent of the parent and child profiles is to make parents more cognizant of the "fit" between their own and their child's characteristics and to note where conflicts between them may arise. Also, parents may strive to modify their own characteristics, where possible, or at least keep them from exacerbating management problems with the child by bearing them in mind. Just as reviewing the child's characteristics with the family may suggest that the family's conflict with this child is not entirely the parents' fault, so this review of parent characteristics may suggest that such conflict is not entirely the child's fault either.

Situational Consequences

Among the most important factors contributing to child behavioral disorders are the consequences for families when the child behaves inappropriately. In fact, it is through these consequences, particularly those provided by the parents, that several of the other factors described in this model operate. It appears that parent characteristics and family stress events operate directly on the ability of parents to provide consistent, appropriate, and effective consequences during the management of child behavior. In addition, child characteristics certainly affect the manner in which the child reacts to these management efforts and hence indirectly affect the consequences the parents will subsequently employ to deal with the child's reactions.

Describe for the parents the notion that children do not behave without cause or reason— that is, child behavior is not random but occurs because of particular response predispositions of the child (the characteristics described above), his/her learning history within the family, and the consequences occurring in the immediate situation in which the problem behavior arises. The processes whereby these consequences operate can be subdivided into two fundamental concepts: positive reinforcement and escape/avoidance learning (negative reinforcement). These processes were discussed in Chapter 1 of this manual and should be discussed now with the parents in language that is readily understandable to them.

Essentially, parents are taught that children may misbehave to gain positive consequences or rewards, or to escape from currently ongoing unpleasant, boring, or effortful activities. Parents are asked to describe the types of positive consequences that may accrue to children for misbehavior. Most parents are quite capable of providing a rather accurate list of such consequences. They appear to have somewhat greater difficulty generating a list of consequences children might wish to avoid, and so your assistance here may be necessary. Point out to parents that most of the activities we assign children to do, especially chores, are not especially pleasant, often require extended effort, and require the child to stop what he/she was doing (usually something enjoyable) to perform this unpleasant activity. As a result, children may experiment with ways of escaping from or avoiding chores by developing oppositional behavior toward parent commands. You will find it helpful to show the schematic diagram of an oppositional–defiant interaction from Chapter 1 (see Figure 1.2), and so it is provided for you to photocopy in Part IV of this manual. Describe it in some detail so parents can appreciate how consequences they are providing for oppositional behavior are serving to create and sustain it, typically through the children's periodic success at escaping unwanted activities parents wish to impose on them.

Explain that a child need not be successful all the time in gaining positive consequences or avoiding unpleasant activities in order to show disruptive, noncompliant, or oppositional behavior to most commands. This is the principle of intermittent reinforcement and, as most therapists know, such partial schedules of consequences can strengthen and sustain noncompliance in children even though the child succeeds with such behavior only a minority of the time. The terminology of behavioral psychology, as noted earlier, is not helpful to use with families; instead, use lay language and stress that periodic success by the child can play a role in maintaining his/her defiance. Sometimes using the example of adult gambling and how it is maintained by small periodic payoffs helps to convey this notion to parents. Again, teaching the jargon is not so important as conveying the concept to the parents.

Family Stress Events

Now you should review with the parents a variety of potential stress events that families may experience. These can be subdivided into stressors related to personal problems, the marital relationship, health problems, financial problems, one or both spouses' occupations, problems with relatives and friends, and problems created by siblings in the family.

Parents should be taught that these stress events can act in several ways to increase the likelihood of noncompliant or inappropriate behavior in children. First, because they directly affect the parents' own emotional well-being, they will certainly affect how effectively and consistently parents will deal with unacceptable behavior when it occurs. Parents may fluctuate in their management tactics much more so when under stress. They may increase their commands, supervision, and punishment of a child because of their own irritable mood. Alternatively some may withdraw from managing the child's behavior, due to preoccupation with the stress events and the anxiety and depression that may accompany them. Either way, parental management of children becomes far more variable and inconsistent, leading to greater success of child oppositional behavior in escaping or avoiding unpleasant or effortful tasks.

A second way in which family stress affects child misbehavior is by altering parental perceptions of the child. Depressed, anxious, or distressed parents tend to exaggerate their reports of child behavior problems. That is, such parents perceive the child's misbehavior as being more severe than it is because it is more distressing for them, given their own mental status. Should parents act on these perceptions, which they typically do, then they will behave toward the child as if his/her behavior were deviant or unacceptable when in fact it is not. In so doing, parents may inadvertently punish normal or acceptable child behavior; increase their commands, directiveness, and general negativism toward children; and begin using negative words to describe the child's character or personality, which can affect not only child behavior but also self-esteem. In short, they may overreact to garden-variety child misconduct. This may then lead to deviant behavior by the child where none previously existed, confirming the parents' initial perception that the child was deviant.

A third way in which family stress increases misbehavior in children is by its direct effects on the child and his/her own emotional well-being. Like the parents, children can become preoccupied with family stress events, and these can create anxiety, depression, or distress. These may then heighten the child's likelihood of displaying negative, oppositional, or noncompliant behavior.

You must help parents appreciate the role of family stress in creating or exacerbating child misbehavior. Marital discord, family financial troubles, tense relations with relatives, and so forth, can all create an emotional climate in the home in which child oppositional behavior may flourish, in part because stress affects the manner in which parents both percieve and deal with everyday child management problems. Certainly, the parents cannot be expected to solve all of the potential stress events impinging upon them immediately, but they should be encouraged to begin making plans for how they intend to reduce the stress created by a particular family situation. Many times, parents simply choose to accept their fate and live with whatever stressors may be occurring, even though efforts can be made to try to resolve them. At the very least, parents need to become aware that such stressors are affecting their management of the child and take steps to see that they buffer the child from such an influence. To assist with initiating this process, parents can either complete the Family Problems Inventory (provided in Part IV of this manual, for photocopying) during the session or it can be assigned as homework, should the training format be a parent group. In either case this form is completed so the parent may take stock of potential stressors and start proposing solutions to them where feasible.

The Reciprocal Interaction among These Factors

You should now briefly explain to the parents that, while each of these factors contributes directly to creating or sustaining noncompliant behavior in children, they can also influence each of the other factors, resulting in even further difficulties in the family. For instance, medical problems with either a parent or a child can influence the family financial situation, which itself may then affect the parents' marital relationship. This feeds back to exacerbate child misbehavior. These interactions can create a veritable cauldron of risk events within families that may foment even greater behavioral problems with the child over time.

The Goal of Therapy: Engineering a "Best Fit"

At this point, it is helpful to summarize the foregoing presentation by saying that many times the characteristics of the parent or child are such that they will naturally prove irritating to the other. Similarly, certain parent or child characteristics may not react well to certain family stress events, which only bring out the deviant parent or child characteristic further and increase deviant behavior in both parties. One goal of therapy is to try to change these poorly fitting situational, parental, and child characteristics where possible so as to lessen the behavioral problems of the child. This can be achieved through showing parents how to do the following:

1. Recognize their own "risk" factors, change them where possible, or at least try to prevent these factors from interfering with their effective management of their child.

2. Recognize certain "risk" factors in the child, attempt to change them where feasible, and at least learn to accept those that cannot be changed and strive to cope with them as possible.

3. Change the situational consequences they are providing for child noncompliance that often serve to create, maintain, or exacerbate defiant child behavior.

The Need for a Prosthetic Social Environment

For parents of children having mild behavior problems or oppositional behavior, it is very possible that this program will bring their child's behavior back within the normally accepted range of social conduct. In other words, the problems for which the family sought help can be "cured." However, with more serious behavioral problems, such as those experienced by children with ADHD, pervasive developmental disorders, psychosis, or other such developmental disorders, this parent training program will not "cure" the disorders. Instead, they will greatly reduce the distress the parents experience over the child's disruptive, noncompliant, and generally unacceptable behavior as well as reducing the child's defiant behavior. In such cases, parent training can create a long-term, ongoing, prosthetic social environment for the children that maximizes their ability to behave appropriately. Even at their best, such children will certainly have more difficulties with familial and social conduct than normal children. But they need not experience the level of deviant behavior often seen at the time of referral. A corollary of this is that such children need these methods if they are to do what normal children appear to be able to accomplish without such professional help. Like a mechanical prosthetic limb, these behavior management techniques will serve to permit the behaviorally handicapped child to become more normal. Remove the prosthetic techniques and the child may well revert to previous and higher levels of deviant behavior. Unlike the mechanical limb, however, it may be possible gradually to reduce the frequency, intensity, and systematic usage of these behavioral methods over long time intervals as the child matures and gains greater self-control, such that the gains of therapy are eventually maintained.

Tailor the above explanation of these issues as they apply to the particular child, parent, and family circumstances of each case. A strong emphasis should be placed at this time on the critical role that parental motivation plays in the success of this treatment program. No matter how effective these techniques have proven with others, they will not help the parents unless the methods are used. Stress that you cannot do it for the parents; they must practice and implement the procedures themselves if any real hope of changing the child is to be realized. Some parents approach therapy for their child with the attitude that it is the therapist's job, and not their own, to change their child for the better. This is a "Jiffy Lube" approach to child therapy wherein the parents view their role as simply dropping off the child with a mental health professional, who will fix the child's problems while they sit in a waiting room. Such a parental attitude obviously is counterproductive and needs to be addressed head on, if necessary, at this early stage of therapy.

Homework

There are two homework assignments for this session. First, the parents are to complete the Family Problems Inventory over the next week if it was not completed during the session. Encourage each parent to complete one separately. The parents need not share their answers with each other if they so choose, but where this lack of sharing occurs, it is obvious evidence of marital disharmony and should be duly noted by the therapist. The parent is to list briefly the stress events occurring under each category and then briefly propose what, if anything, he/she intends to do about them. Parents do not have to solve their problems this week, but they should at least formulate plans to reduce those stressors noted. I am often surprised to find that material is divulged on the inventory that was not previously revealed in the initial evaluation of the family, now that the parents can appreciate the role of such stressors in child misbehavior. For families receiving training in a group, you should state that the contents of their inventory will not be shared with the rest of the parent group when it is turned in at the next class. Instead, you will review it privately and speak with the parents about any significant stressors that may deserve more immediate attention. Occasionally, something is revealed that results in training being temporarily postponed while that issue is addressed.

The second assignment is to have the parents childproof their home, if they have not already done so. Research indicates that oppositional children, especially those with comorbid ADHD, are more accident prone, more likely to damage property and valuables, and more likely to create accidents for others than are normal children. Parents should be encouraged to review each room in their home for potentially harmful agents or machines, for valuable property that could inadvertently be damaged by the young child, or for items that the parents wish to preserve or protect that are now within easy reach of the impulsive child.

Pay Attention!

Goals

1. To educate parents about how the style of their interactions with their children greatly affects their children's motivation to work for them.

2. To train parents in methods of attending to positive child behavior while differentially ignoring negative behavior.

3. To require parents to practice these differential attending skills at home over the next week.

4. To begin establishing a more positive interaction pattern between parent and child.

Materials Required

- Parent Handout for Step 2

  Paying Attention to Your Child's Good Play Behavior

Step Outline

- Review homework

  Family Problems Inventory
  Childproofing the home

- Introduce the rationale for developing attending skills

  Discuss importance of quality of attention to people
  Present "worst" versus "best" supervisor vignette
  Extend discussion to how parents attend to problem child

- Distribute and review parent handout on attending skills

  Review goals of this session
  Stress important features of the skills in the handout
  Discuss parental reactions to the technique

- Model the technique for the parents
- Have parents practice methods in session (if not in group training)
- Determine when "special time" will be done at home

Homework

- Begin daily "special time" practice periods
- Record information on practice of "special time" at home

This session begins with a review of the previous session's homework assignments and whether problems were encountered in completing the Family Problems Inventory, if it was assigned for homework. You may wish to review the contents of the Family Problems Inventory if the training program is being provided on an individual basis to a family. If it is a parent group, these questionnaires are set aside for later review by you outside of the parent group. You should then determine if the parents made any attempt to childproof their home in the case of the young oppositional child. If neither assignment was given, then proceed to the presentation of the new material for this session.

Introducing the Rationale for Developing Attending Skills

Do not provide the parents with the handout for this session until discussion has occurred on the quality of attention and how it affects people's behavior. Parents should initially be questioned as to whether they believe receiving attention from others is valuable to them. This should then lead to a discussion of how the quality of the attention we receive from others, even as adults, affects our subsequent desire to work them.

In making this presentation, I have found the following technique particularly useful. I ask parents to put aside for the moment any thoughts about their children and instead concentrate on individuals with whom they have worked in the past. Specifically, parents are asked to think about the worst person with whom they have ever worked, usually a supervisor, and to try to describe the characteristics of that person that led to those feelings. It is helpful here to have the parents divide a sheet of paper in half with a line running vertically down the page. At the top of the left-hand column, they should write the heading "Worst Supervisor." In this column, they are to write at least five characteristics of the worst person with whom they have worked. If this is a parent group, use a blackboard and record the answers given by all parents on the board. Parents usually have little difficulty thinking of these characteristics, but if they should, assistance can be provided. Time should be taken to get the parents to specify the feelings they had toward this person because of these undesirable ways in which they were treated. In particular, you are trying to get parents to acknowledge that the manner in which they were treated affected their motivation to work for this supervisor and probably the quality of their own work for this person.

After these characteristics are discussed, have the parents write the heading "Best Supervisor" at the top of the right-hand column. Parents are then instructed to imagine the best person with whom they have worked. They subsequently are to record at least five characteristics about the person that made them feel this way. These responses are recorded in the right-hand column of the paper. Again, answers from parents in a parent training group can be recorded on a blackboard. Here the therapist is attempting to get parents to articulate how this optimal treatment by a supervisor increased their motivation to work for this person and probably raised the quality of that work as well.

At this point, the connection of this vignette to the purposes of the training program can be made obvious to the parents. This is done simply by asking the parents which of these two columns, or which of these two supervisors, they are most similar to in their own interactions with the behavior problem child. Most parents honestly report that they are more often like the "worst" supervisor than the "best" supervisor in this exercise. Time should be taken to discuss how their child might come to feel about working for the parents as the parents did about working for such a "worst" supervisor. It is possible that the child may have, in a behavioral sense, gone "on strike" or created a "work slowdown" in their work at home for their parents because of the poor quality of parental supervision and work conditions in the home.

Discussing the Objectives of the Session

Having introduced the notion that the quality of our work for others and the way we feel about them is greatly determined by the way in which they interacted with or "attended" to us, you should now review the objectives of this session with the parents. Primary among these is the need, hopefully demonstrated in the exercise above, to improve the quality of parental attention given to the defiant child. Granted, improving that attention is unlikely to be sufficient to ameliorate the problems with this child completely, but it is a necessary first step in that process. In addition, as noted earlier, the reward value to children of parental attention in families with behavior problem children is generally lower than that in normal families. Hence, if parental attention is to be used to improve child compliance, it must first be enhanced in value. The methods to be introduced here will contribute to that goal.

A second purpose of this session is to improve the general relations occurring between parent and child through the use of the nondirective "attending" practice periods to be done for homework. This leads the child to feel that the parents are interested in him/her, despite the fact that the child may have behaved badly during the day. This practice is done in order to reverse the progressive trend often seen in such families where the parents often spend less time in leisure activities with the problem child. In other words, the play procedures in this session are designed to get parents and children interacting more positively toward each other more often than was previously the case. Many parents report a renewed sense of pleasure in playing with the child following these guidelines, and I believe the children come to feel the same, given their frequent requests for additional such play periods once they are begun. Although such a goal may seem overly ambitious to parents at this stage of training, it is often noted at the end of even 1 week of conducting these "special" playtimes that the parents in fact find the children more desirable persons with whom to interact and vice versa.

A third objective of this step is to get parents to begin differentially attending to positive child behaviors while ignoring negative ones. This is often contrary to the parents' current practice of ignoring positive child behaviors while attending or responding only to the disruptive or negative ones. Each of these objectives should be described to the parents to ensure that they fully understand the rationale for the play technique to be discussed in the parent handout.

Reviewing the Parent Handout

The handout for Step 2 should now be distributed for the parents to read. Afterward, review the important points of the handout in some detail. As the handout indicates, this session is designed to train parents in using new methods of paying attention to child behaviors during play. The handout instructs parents to select a time when the child is playing in an activity that the child normally enjoys and that is appropriate. Parents are then to approach the child and begin a period of 15–20 minutes of playing with him/her in the manner discussed in the handout. Parents are encouraged to make this "special time" an even more formal activity by telling the child that the parent will henceforth be taking time each day to play with him/her. The child is then asked what activity he/she would like to do around the home that day for the special time. The child is permitted to choose the activity, within reason. It is essential that the child selects the activity so that he/she comes to believe that the parents are interested in what he/she wants to do and not in simply taking charge of the play and redirecting it to something that the parents desire to do.

As suggested in the handout, it is critical that the parents learn to relax during this time, and that the parents have absolutely nothing else on their minds other than learning to attend to what the child is doing. For this reason, parents should not attempt to play with the child immediately before going out on an errand or shopping trip as it is likely that the quality of the attention provided by the parent would be quite superficial. It is the sole purpose of this playtime to practice attending positively to ongoing child behaviors.

During the playtime, the parents should watch, mentally note, and follow the child's various activities for a few moments before beginning to narrate what the child is doing. This narrative description should occur occasionally throughout the playtime. By doing so, the child will begin to develop the idea that the parents are quite interested in what he/she does, regardless of how trivial or simple it may seem at the time. In addition, the narration of the child's activities necessarily precludes the parents from asking intrusive questions or giving commands in such a way that they come to take charge of the play activities. As noted in the handout, parents are to avoid giving any commands or asking questions during this time where possible.

One method for teaching parents to adopt this style of narration is to have them imagine being a sportscaster describing the action of a sporting event for a radio broadcast. The description should be interesting, detailed, and generally a running, uncritical commentary on the events taking place. Depending on the way in which the parents choose to narrate and the degree to which this narration is embellished with cues of interest and excitement, this style of paying attention to child behavior can be highly effective at reinforcing children for appropriate play activities. I have found that younger children appreciate this narrative more than older children, who come to find it disruptive of their play activities and somewhat condescending. Parents should therefore exercise their judgment as to how much narration to employ with a child. The important point here, regardless of the child's age, is to have the parents spend time with the child without criticizing, directing, or controlling the child's behavior, instead watching and appreciating what the child does.

As noted above, it is essential that the parents limit their questioning and eliminate any commands that may be given during this time. Commands are obviously designed to take control over an activity, and such control is to be inhibited during the child's playtime. Parents should be told that there is virtually nothing that they need to teach during this playtime that could not be deferred for teaching during some other time. Even if the child's play is not up to the standards expected by the parents, the parents should avoid taking charge of the play and trying to teach the child different ways of playing.

Questions, like commands, are to be avoided as much as possible as they also intrude upon children's play; they necessitate that the children redirect their activities in order to respond to the parents. Older children may require somewhat more questioning during these play activities and may not find it as intrusive as younger children. Furthermore, the kinds of questions asked of younger children are often superfluous because the parent often knows the answer already but is using the question to "quiz" children as to how much they have learned in their development so far. In short, what few questions may be uttered by parents are to be of the more conversational, "cocktail party" sort that express interest in another person and their activities, not of the type that quiz or test the child's knowledge.

Throughout the playtime, the parents should intersperse various comments of positive, genuine feedback. As noted in the handout, this feedback is not necessarily glowing praise for what the child is doing. Instead, it is simply a statement that reflects the parents' interest in what the child is doing and perhaps the parents' enjoyment of being with the child. A list of positive phrases that parents may use during play appears on the last page of the handout for Step 2. I include this list in the handout so that parents do not come to use only one or two well-worn phrases of appreciation during this special playtime. Parents are taught that positive feedback can be given not only verbally, but also through physical gestures that communicate approval and appreciation. Praise, when given, should be quite specific and can emphasize not only what the child is doing that is acceptable, but also what he/she is not doing that was previously unacceptable. Parents should be quite specific as to the behavior they are appreciating rather than utilizing vague references, such as "good boy" or "nice girl." I believe that such specificity increases the effectiveness of praise as a reinforcer for a child's behavior.

Many parents ask at this point how they should behave during the special playtime if their child begins to become seriously disruptive. It is my belief that the parents' best reaction is simply to turn away momentarily from the child in an effort to ignore the problem behavior. Often, this readily reduces it. Should the unacceptable behavior escalate, however, the parents should merely tell the child that the special time has ended and that it can resume again later once the child is behaving appropriately. On rare occasions, the level of misbehavior will be such that it is deserving of punishment. At this point, the parents are instructed to handle the disciplining in a manner similar to the way in which they have been handling it previously. No effort should be made here to introduce the methods of discipline to be taught later in this program, such as time out from reinforcement. Parents should be told that misbehavior during special time is quite rare in our experience. This probably has to do with the fact that no commands are being given to the child, and these often serve as prompts to the child to misbehave or act in an oppositional manner.

You should note that the special playtime is to be conducted alone with the defiant child, without siblings or the spouse interfering. If necessary, such special time can be given to the other children in the family at another time of day, but the time with the problem child is always to be on a one-to-one basis. This precludes the problem child having to share his/her special playtime with siblings whose behaviors and characteristics may be more desirable than his/her own and hence more likely to draw parental praise and attention away from the problem child. Where two parents are present, one can take the siblings away to another room for activities while the second practices the special attending methods during play with the problem child. After 15–20 minutes, the parents can change their respective roles, giving each spouse a chance to practice these attending skills. If not convenient for the second parent at that time, then a separate special time should be scheduled for this parent to practice with the problem child as well.

Common Parental Reactions to the Methods

Parents should be provided ample time to discuss any of their concerns about or reactions to this method. Often, parents note that they have not had time to do such playing with the child since the birth of younger siblings into the family. Parents commonly remark at this point that the play techniques seem especially simple and will be quite easy to implement. Such is not the case, as noted at the bottom of the handout. Inhibiting commands and questions, concentrating on positive narration, and providing occasional positive feedback take considerable practice to do well. The elimination of commands and questions is quite difficult for many parents, as they are accustomed to controlling their children's behavior much of the day via these mechanisms. Parents often find themselves at a loss for what to say during playtime once these social devices have been forbidden by the therapist. Instruction can be provided on ways of translating questions into comments or reflective remarks by parents.

Another reaction often heard from parents is that the special time does not seem directed at the problems of the child for which they sought treatment. Hopefully, this issue will have been handled by the exercise at the beginning of the session comparing qualities of "best" versus "worst" supervisors. If not, then you can reiterate here the need for parents to improve the quality and value of their attending skills with children before such attention can be used to increase child compliance to commands. The need to rebuild the parent–child relationship should be made obvious. The fact that this method can contribute to that process is often supported by the observation that most children so treated have requested that the playtime continue beyond its usual stopping point—clearly a sign that the child finds the parents' newly developing attending skills to be quite reinforcing.

Some parents comment that if they spend special time with the children that is filled with praise and appreciation, the children will come to expect such treatment for everything they do. There are several ways to handle such remarks. First, it can be pointed out that this has not happened with the thousands of families treated under this program to date. Second, it is helpful to explore with the parents the basis for this attitude toward child behaviors. Obviously, the parents are being paid by an employer for their own work, which is in a sense a similar way of reinforcing them for their performance on the job. Without such payment, few parents would return to work. Furthermore, most parents expect a certain amount of gratitude from their employers, spouses, as well as older children, for the everyday responsibilities the parent handles for these other people. Like the child, they too desire the appreciation and recognition of others for what they do within their employment settings, family, or even community activities. In short, the child desires attention the same way parents do. You can note here that many marriages have foundered because one spouse felt "taken for granted," which is merely another way of saying that their contributions to the marriage were unappreciated.

Some parents may note that they are too busy for this sort of activity. The remark conveys the essence of an important problem in such families—that there is little time or importance assigned to childrearing. Is it any wonder behavior problems in the children have emerged from such a family interaction pattern? I have sometimes responded to such remarks, half humorously, by suggesting that the parents consider placing the child up for adoption if they are unable to find even 15 minutes in their day for practicing such special attention to a child.

Modeling and Practicing the Methods

If the training is provided in a single-family format and the child is available during the session, you can take the child to a corner of the room and begin playing with the child such that the parents can observe these activities. The therapist models the appropriate methods, taking care to make an occasional mistake that can then be discussed with the parents later in the session. Resources permitting, a therapist may wish to videotape such a play session with a child to show to other parents undergoing training in this session. Thereafter, the parents should practice the attending skills with their child in front of the therapist, with appropriate feedback being provided by the therapist. Afterward, the parents should review with you the feelings they have about these methods. Many parents report that they found the attending to be more difficult in practice than they initially believed it would be when hearing it described.

In the case of parent training groups, it is not possible for the parents to practice with their own child. Some therapists might wish to have parents pair off and role play, where one parent pretends to be the child while the other practices giving this type of special attention. This role playing may prove impractical, however. In my experience, discussion of the method with parents in a training group, along with the parental handout for this session, is often sufficient for them to get the gist of what they are to practice at home.

Parents should then discuss how they intend to implement the daily special times at home during the coming week(s). They should be encouraged to choose a particular time of day that is best for both parent and child, perhaps when other siblings are occupied with their own activities. Where possible, each parent is to practice the attending skills daily with the child. For older children, it may not be as helpful to have a formal time set aside each day, because such children may often be involved with various out-of-home activities or school homework. In such cases, parents should watch throughout the day for times that seem opportune to approach and interact with the child over some play activity in which the child is currently engaged. Watching television together is discouraged because verbal narration or discussion during that activity is often annoying or intrusive.

If the child chooses a competitive game, parents should allow the child to invent new rules or even "cheat" in the game without recrimination during this playtime. Parents should remember that the purpose of the time is not to learn how to play a game properly, but to practice their own attending skills toward the child. Nonetheless, cooperative games and activities lend themselves better to this special time than do competitive ones.

Care should be taken to explain to the parents that this special playtime is not going to miraculously cure all of the child's behavioral problems. In fact, noncompliance by the child during the subsequent week is often unabated because it is mostly in reaction to parental commands rather than such special play periods. What the parents can expect, however, is that the child may come to view the parents as more desirable people with whom to interact and work. Although this may not occur for some families, most report a slight improvement in their relationship with the child after only 1 week. Parents should also be told that this special playtime is to become a part of the household routine for an indefinite period of time. After the first week of practice, the parents can reduce the frequency of special time with the child to three or four times per week but should strive to maintain this frequency indefinitely throughout the childhood years, tapering it down as the child enters adolescence.

Homework

Parents are then instructed in the homework for the coming week. Parents are to practice the attending skills during special time on a daily basis, where possible, for the coming week. They should record a few sentences in a notebook as to what they did during each day's special time and how the child reacted. Parents may wish to note special problems they encountered with the methods to discuss during the next training session. With this assigned as homework, parents are more likely to practice the procedures because they are more accountable for their week's activities with the child.

Increasing Compliance and Independent Play

Goals

1. To train parents to use effective attending skills to increase immediate child compliance with parental commands.

2. To increase the effectiveness of parental commands in eliciting child compliance.

3. To increase the use by parents of effective attending skills for independent, nondisruptive compliance by children.

4. To increase parental monitoring of child behavior in the home and neighborhood.

Materials Required

- Parent Handouts for Step 3

    Paying Attention to Your Child's Compliance
    Giving Effective Commands
    Attending to Independent Play

Step Outline

- Review homework

    Parents' use of special attending skills
    Reminder to continue "special time" periods with child

- Explain extension of attending skills from play to compliance
- Review ways of increasing effectiveness of commands
- Discuss use of compliance training periods at home
- Discuss with parents how children disrupt their activities
- Distribute parent handout on decreasing disruption and increasing independent play

- Modeling of methods by therapist
- Review parental reactions to methods
- Instruct parents to increase monitoring of child behavior

Homework

- Continue "special time" periods with child
- Begin praising and attending to compliance
- Establish daily compliance training periods
- Give effective commands
- Practice attending to independent play
- Increase monitoring of children's independent activities

The parents' records of their special playtime activities should be reviewed. If parents are in individual family training and failed to do the assignment, no new material is presented. Instead, the reason for this failure is addressed and the parents are requested to try it again during the coming week. If the parents are in group training, this failure is duly noted and a separate session with the parents is to be scheduled outside of group training to review the matter privately with them. These procedures for dealing with homework noncompliance were discussed earlier and are to be used whenever homework is not done. They, therefore, will not be repeated in the discussion of subsequent sessions. Otherwise, for parents completing the homework, you should instruct the parents that they are to continue the "special playtimes" with the child indefinitely on a frequency of three to four times per week. This will (1) produce further improvements in the parent–child relationship; (2) allow the child to continue to receive moments of positive attention from parents despite what, at times, may be a day filled with difficult child behavior; and (3) build child self-esteem.

Some parents comment that their children appeared to be both pleasantly surprised and dismayed at the new attention they were receiving from their parents. A few children may have even questioned the parents as to a hidden motive for this unexpected positive attention. After the initial surprise has passed, many children settle easily into the routine of the daily special playtimes, often reminding their parents of the commitment should the parents forget. Many of the children request that the playtime continue beyond its normal 15- to 20-minute limit. A few parents seem pleasantly surprised that their children find them to be so desirable after years of oppositional behavior and arguments from the children. Some parents will have found no change in their children's behavior. They should be told not to be discouraged as the method may take longer to yield benefits for some children, especially if the history of negative parent–child relations has been a long and difficult one for both parties. A few parents complain that while the children appeared to enjoy the play periods, they did not expressly thank the parents for having taken the time to be with them. These parents should be instructed that the important thing is that the children received the attention, not that the children expressly acknowledge it. The true impact of the play period will be judged in the weeks to come as a result of its effects on the parents' own attending skills and on the parent–child relationship.

Extending the Attending Skills from Play to Compliance

Provide the parents with the first handout for this session. The handout is brief and should be easily understood by most parents. Essentially, parents are to "catch their children being good" and to respond to compliance with attention, appreciation, and praise. The purpose of the session is to teach parents to increase compliance with commands by providing positive consequences, in this case parental attention, contingent upon child compliance with commands. Parents are instructed to pay particular attention this week to when they issue commands to their children. At these times, they are to remain in the area where compliance is to be carried out, watch, narrate, and appreciate the compliant activities of the child. In many cases, parents issue commands and then depart the area to attend to other matters, returning periodically to see if the task has been done. In this session, parents are taught to remain near the child during compliance so as to provide ongoing positive attention and comments about the child's compliance. Statements of praise and appreciation should be quite specific as to what the parents find positive in the child's behavior, such as "I like it when you do as I say," or "Mom really likes it when you pick up your toys." Parents usually have little difficulty understanding this concept. However, actually increasing their praise of child compliance is another matter and will take practice.

Parents should be instructed to provide particularly salient positive attention and rewards to a child who has complied with a household rule or routine chore without having been instructed to do so, particularly when the child previously was noncompliant with that rule or chore. It is believed that this increases the likelihood of the child internalizing such rules and routines and complying with them in future situations.

Giving Effective Commands

You can now provide the second handout for this session, which deals with methods for improving the effectiveness of parental commands. These are straightforward recommendations, which can be briefly commented on by the therapist. First, the parents should be sure that they mean the command they are about to give and are willing to see the task to its completion. Second, the command should be presented as a direct statement, not a favor or a question. It need not be presented in a negative tone of voice, but it should be clear to the child that the parent is serious about the task. Third, parents should give simple commands rather than multiple ones when dealing with the behavior disordered child. Adequate time should be allotted to see that the first request has been obeyed before issuing a subsequent command. Fourth, parents should make eye contact with the child. Yelling out commands to a child from an adjoining room is not helpful. Parents should look directly at the child to ensure his/her undivided attention, especially where children have comorbid ADHD. Fifth, parents should reduce significant distractors in the area before initiating a command. For instance, if the child is watching television, playing a video game, or listening to a stereo system, the parent should either first instruct the child to turn the apparatus off or the parent should do so before assigning the task to be done. Parents are unlikely to have much success competing with these highly stimulating and engaging devices. Sixth, where necessary, have the child repeat the command back to the parent to ensure he/she has understood the request and to reinforce his/her memory of the command. Finally, parents may wish to assign time limits and create "chore cards" for extended tasks, such as cleaning a bedroom or doing homework. For the former, the parents should set a specified time on a kitchen timer and let the child know the time limits and consequences. For the latter, the parents can write down the series of steps in such a protracted task, so that the child can carry the card with him/her during the performance of the job. Using such "chore cards" ensures that there can be no debate from the child over what the components were in the task.

Establishing Compliance Training Periods

In teaching any new behavior or increasing the occurrence of one already present in a child's repertoire, the rate of acquisition or the increase in the desired behavior is related to the number of training opportunities available for reinforcing that behavior. In view of this principle, I have found it useful to have parents actually increase their rate of commands to a child during a brief training period so as to permit more opportunities for reinforcing compliance to requests. These compliance training periods should last about 3–5 minutes, and parents should have at least two or three each day. During these periods, parents should ask the child to perform a series of simple requests, each of which requires minimal effort by the child, such as "Hand me that magazine," "Come here and let me tuck in your shirt/blouse," "Please get me the salt shaker," and so forth. Such commands are less likely to meet with oppositional behavior because they involve minimal work by the children. Parents are then to use this time expressly to attend to, praise, and otherwise reward the child for compliance. For very young children, a small taste of a favorite snack food or drink can be given during this time for compliance to some of the commands. For older children, appreciation will be sufficient for now. Parents should implement these training periods at times of the day when the child is not engaged in some special or desirable activity but appears to be between play activities, as this is likely to increase the probability of compliance.

You should model the methods for the parents and then review the parents' reactions to them before proceeding to teach the next procedure in this session. If training is being done with an individual family, this modeling by the therapist can, once again, be done with the child to allow parents to observe the therapist using these techniques. Subsequently, the parents practice them in the therapist's presence. In group training, the modeling of the methods by the therapist followed by group discussion is sufficient.

Common Parent Reactions to the Methods

1. *What if the child fails to comply with my commands during this week?* Tell parents to handle the child's noncompliance as they typically have done. You are not yet ready to teach parents the disciplining procedures of this program, so do not get lulled into training discipline methods before the other steps have been mastered.

2. *What if the child does not comply with the commands I give during the special compliance training periods?* Tell parents simply to ignore the noncompliance for the moment and issue another brief command for the child to do something else for the parent.

3. *Praise has never motivated my child. Why should I expect it to work this week?* Although not as common as the other parental reactions noted here, this reaction sometimes occurs and often shows that the parent has not fully appreciated the lesson from Step 2—that some types of praise and attention are more valuable to children than others. It is likely that the parents have previously employed ineffective attending and praising skills; certainly they are unlikely to have used them in the style being taught in this program. You can respond to these parents by indicating that the praise and attention you are asking that they try is likely to be different from what they have used previously and therefore may now result in motivating their child. Even then, changing a child's behavior may take more than just 1 week of parental praising of the child, and so patience is required. Finally, such praise and attention will slowly begin to improve child self-esteem even though the changes in compliance are not dramatic or immediate. Such change in child self-esteem is a laudable goal in itself.

4. *Isn't giving commands in this way too harsh?* Some parents believe that giving commands as imperatives violates etiquette; it lacks the courtesy of the favors, requests, and other social niceties that are commonly used when asking others to do things for us. Although such etiquette may be used with normally well-behaved children, it is highly unlikely to elicit compliance from clinic-referred defiant children when used by their parents. You should inform parents of this, saying that when the children become compliant, parents can return to using such social graces for the purpose of teaching proper etiquette. For now, it is essential that children first learn to comply with parental authority. This is not to say that parents cannot preface their commands and directives with the word "please," only that such directives not be issued as requests for favors, such as "Why don't you pick up the toys now, okay?" The latter form of a "command favor" has been shown in research to be much less likely to elicit compliance from oppositional children.

Discussing Disruptive Behavior by Children

Before distributing the third handout for this session, the therapist should engage the parents in a discussion of the specific kinds of disruptive behavior often seen in their child and the parents' beliefs about why this behavior persists. Parents often report that they are unable to talk on the telephone, speak with visitors in the home or with their spouse in the evening, read newspapers or magazines, or otherwise engage in a task without the behavior problem child disrupting them. Many parents will note that children do so in an effort to gain attention from parents, and this is certainly the case. But if parental attention is such a motivator of children's disruptive behavior, then why don't children resist bothering their parents in order to get attention? This question should be posed to parents because its answer is obvious: There is minimal attention paid in this family to children when they are playing or complying independently of their parents and not disrupting parental activities.

This situation is easily illustrated by using the example of talking on the telephone. Most parents of behavior problem children describe this situation as highly problematic for them due to child disruptiveness. The parents should be asked if they have ever temporarily interrupted their telephone conversation to yell at, reprimand, or discipline a child for disruption. Most, if not all, will answer in the affirmative. Then parents should be asked whether they have ever interrupted their conversation to praise or attend to a child for *not* disrupting the call but instead playing quietly nearby. Few, if any, parents will answer yes to such a question. The implication of this situation is that if children wish to receive parental attention, they are most successful at doing so through disruption of parental activities, particularly if that activity involves attention being paid to someone else other than the child. Clearly, if the situation were reversed and parental attention were given for nondisruptive behavior, then children should decrease their disruptiveness and increase their playing independently of their parents.

Distributing and Explaining the Independent Play Handout

At this point, the parents should be provided with the third handout for this session, dealing with Attending to Independent Play. Afterwards, explain the method described in the handout, which is essentially a shaping procedure. The method involves having the parent initially attend to a child's nondisruptive behavior on a very frequent basis. Then the frequency of attention is gradually reduced as the child spends longer periods of time not disrupting the parent while the parent is busy. When disruptions do occur, they are to be ignored by the parent as much as possible.

You can illustrate the method by an example of a parent trying to read a magazine or cook a meal. In either case, the parent should always begin by assigning the child some desirable activity to perform while the parent is busy, or to at least stipulate that the child is not to bother the parent. For instance, the parent might say, "I want you to sit here and color in your book while I read this magazine. Do not interrupt me." The parent then begins reading the magazine but stops within a minute or so to praise the child for complying and not bothering her. The command is then reissued to the child and the mother resumes reading. She then reads for a slightly longer interval, stopping again to praise the child for compliance. She returns to reading, this time for an even longer interval, after which the child is praised. Gradually, the intervals of reading are progressively lengthened before the parent provides further praise and attention to the child. For very young children, small tastes of a favorite snack food can be used periodically to reinforce independent play.

A similar progression might be seen if the mother were attempting to prepare a meal. Once again, the child is directed to play away from the mother and assigned a particular play activity (e.g., watch television, color, play with blocks, etc.). The mother then initiates the meal preparation but stops her work frequently to praise the child. The intervals between reinforcements of the child are then gradually lengthened until the child is able to play for 5–10 minutes of sustained, nondisruptive activity (depending on developmental abilities), with parental attention given only at the end of the interval.

This takes some patience and organizational talent by the parents but most can acquire this simple shaping procedure quite easily. Parents should remember that the initial purpose of the activity is not for them to read or cook but to watch and reinforce their child for not bothering them. As they gradually shape up the interval of time the child can play independently, they will then be able to read or perform some other activity uninterrupted.

Modeling and Practicing the Attending to Independent Play

You can now model the method by taking the child to a separate playroom or to a corner of your office where the parent can observe you, as in prior sessions, and instructing the child to play with a toy while you read nearby. The child is told not to interrupt. Because children are more likely to obey you than their parents in such encounters, you should have little difficulty with noncompliance with such a request. You should then sit nearby and read a few lines of a magazine before putting it down, approaching the child, and praising him/her for not interrupting the reading. Then return to reading for a slightly longer time interval, stop again and praise the child for playing alone, and then continue reading. As above, the intervals of reading are then gradually lengthened with occasional reinforcement of the child being provided. The parents are then to practice the procedure with your supervision, if single-family training is the format employed with this family.

Common Parental Reactions to Attending to Independent Play

Parents often have several reactions to this method. First, many parents operate under the philosophy of "let sleeping dogs lie." This translates into simply not paying attention to their children when they are behaving quietly and appropriately for fear that the parent's attention will only spark new occurrences of undesirable behavior. In fact, such parents will often say that they have tried to reward their children previously for appropriate independent play, only to find that their rewards triggered new episodes of aversive or noncompliant behavior. Explain to these parents that when the independent play of their children is not rewarded, there is no reason to expect that it will recur with any greater frequency. In fact, it is likely to diminish over time because of the lack of reinforcement for its occurrence. Furthermore, tell these parents that the children are probably misbehaving when the parents attend to them because the children have learned that this is one method of keeping the parents in the room for greater lengths of time. If the children were to continue to play appropriately, the parents would be likely to leave the room again. Thus, these children have learned that when the parents come to praise them, the best way to sustain that parental attention is to begin to behave inappropriately. The technique taught in this session, by contrast, is simply to reward the children for independent play and to ignore them or leave the room when misbehavior occurs.

A second reaction of parents is that they complain of not being able to finish their own activities if they must interrupt them frequently to attend to the child's independent play. Although this may be true initially, after several days it is quite possible for a child to learn to play independently for increasingly longer periods of time without disturbing the parent. The eventual result is that the child can play alone for the entire time that the parent is involved in his/her own tasks without the need for frequent reinforcement for doing so (within certain developmental limits of children's attention spans). The parents simply have to invest the time in frequent visits to the child initially in order to achieve the eventual goal of having the child play independently of them for sustained periods.

Increasing Parental Monitoring of Children's Activities

Research suggests that inadequate parental monitoring of children's behavior and activities is a major contributor not only to noncompliant and aggressive behavior by children toward others, especially peers and siblings, but also to the development of clandestine antisocial behaviors (Loeber, 1990; Patterson, 1982; Patterson et al., 1992). Covert antisocial behaviors such as stealing, destruction of property, vandalism, and fire setting, as well as lying to avoid detection, seem to flourish when parents fail to monitor the activities of their defiant children adequately, both in and out of the home. This monitoring does not mean constant and proximal supervision of every activity of the child but frequent, periodic checking of the child's activities at random intervals when the child is outside the immediate vicinity of the parent.

You should strongly encourage parents to interrupt their own activities periodically, locate the child, and reward the child for appropriate behavior that has been occurring in the absence of the parent. Such monitoring should be relatively frequent and generally unpredictable from the child's perspective. If the child is found to be misbehaving, swift and appropriate punishment is delivered. One of the greatest difficulties in monitoring child behavior is simply remembering to do so at times when the parent is normally pre-occupied with other tasks. Parents can train themselves to monitor child activities more frequently through the use of simple cooking timers or those on stove or microwave ovens. Set frequently throughout the day to intervals of varying lengths, these timers can alert parents to stop their activities when the alarm is heard and seek out their children. Watches that have hourly chimes or alarms can also be used for this purpose.

Homework

This week parents should try praising and appreciating the child when he/she complies with commands. They should further practice the methods for increasing the effectiveness of their commands and should implement two to three compliance training periods per day. The "special time" activities are to continue but need not be recorded by the parents.

For practicing attending to independent play, parents are instructed to choose one or two occasions when the child often disrupts their activities and to practice this attending procedure at those times. I have found it useful to concentrate initially on situations in the family's home rather than in the homes of others or in public places when practicing this procedure. Parents may wish to use talking on the telephone for practicing the method. If so, I encourage parents to have the spouse or a friend call them daily for the sole purpose of practicing this shaping procedure. This allows the parents to interrupt the call frequently to attend to the child's independent play without being too rude or disruptive to the caller. Gradually, parents will be able to use the method with calls from others to the home without using such frequent reinforcement of the child. Parents should record several sentences each day describing their success or problems in practicing the method. Where two parents are in the home, each should choose a different activity for practice.

Parents should be forewarned that simply increasing attention to compliance and inde-pendent play does not automatically increase compliant behavior or decrease disruptive behavior in all children. For some children, the use of praise may have to be continued over long time periods before it is successful at improving compliance. For others, espe-cially more deviant children, praise may not be sufficient as a reinforcer. Reassure parents that another, more potent reinforcement method will be taught in the next session. For now, they should try to use their praise and attention where possible to encourage compli-ant behavior and improve child self-esteem.

Parents may also need to be reminded to increase their monitoring of their child's activi-ties and behavior if the parents' comments during the evaluation or during treatment sug-gest that such monitoring is less than adequate for a child of his/her age.

When Praise Is Not Enough:
Poker Chips and Points

Goals

1. To establish a formal system that makes child privileges contingent upon child compliance. This is achieved by implementing the home token system.
2. To increase parental attention to and reinforcement of child compliance and appropriate social conduct.
3. To decrease arbitrariness in parental administration of child privileges.

Materials Required

- Home Situations Questionnaire
- Disruptive Behavior Disorders Rating Scale—Parent Form
- Parent Handout for Step 4

    Home Poker Chip/Point System

Step Outline

- Review homework

    Giving effective commands
    Attending to compliance and independent play
    Increasing parental monitoring of child activities

- Reassess child disruptive behavior using rating scales
- Introduce the need for special reward programs
- Explain advantages of a home chip/point system
- Distribute the parent handout

- Establish the token system

     Choosing chips or points
     Making a list of privileges
     Making a list of child target behaviors
     Assigning prices and wages
     Cautions in starting the program

- Discuss parent reactions to the token system

Homework

- Continue previously taught methods

- Implement the chip/point system

- Bring the lists of privileges and jobs to next session

In reviewing the previous week's assignment, you will find that a few parents will have had great success in implementing the skills of attending to children when they were complying with directives or when the children were not disrupting parental work. Other parents may note some improvements but remain unimpressed with the methods, while still others had no success at all. Encourage the parents not to be disheartened, because in the present session they will acquire a very powerful system for increasing child compliance. In fact, my experience has been that over half of the families will report a near complete remission of the child's problem behaviors during the coming week in response to this program. Others will have dramatic success but some behavioral problems will remain. It is the rare family that does not report some improvement in child compliance from the present session, provided they took the time to implement the methods correctly.

Reassessment of Child Disruptive Behavior

As discussed earlier, clinicians need to reassess the child's misbehavior throughout this program. The beginning of this session is a good time to do so. As occurred at the start of Step 1, the therapist should readminister the HSQ and DBDRS-PF (see Part III) to the parents at the beginning of this step. Results can be used to compare with those taken at Step 1. Do not expect much improvement in these ratings over the past three sessions, as the major behavior change techniques have not yet been taught to the parents.

The Need for Special Reward Programs

Scientific research is coming to discover that many clinic-referred children have significant problems with sustained attention, impulsivity, and self-control, which are more likely to be natural characteristics of the child's behavioral and mental abilities than simply learned misbehavior. These children appear to be less sensitive to social praise and attention. As a result, they often do not show improvements in their behavior merely as a function of increasing parental attention to compliance. More powerful reinforcement programs will prove necessary. This can be related to the earlier discussion in Step 1 about children's temperamental characteristics and developmental abilities. In short, some children will simply not perform at normal levels of compliance for mere social praise and attention; more powerful reinforcement systems must be used. For such children, praise is not enough!

It is helpful here to refer back to Step 1 and the idea introduced there that some children, such as those with ADHD, are handicapped in their behavioral control. Such children require prosthetic behavior change methods to permit them to do what other children can do without such formal, artificial, or intense reward programs. Explaining this notion here often addresses a concern voiced by many parents: "Other children do not get such special rewards for doing what they are expected to do, so why should this child?" Clearly the answer is that some children *need* such a systematic reward program where others do not. However, even normal children often improve their behavior under similar poker chip or point systems.

Even in cases where otherwise normal children have oppositional or noncompliant behavior as their only problem, these token systems can result in more rapid behavioral improvements than would have been possible with praise serving as the only reinforcer in the program. Furthermore, such token systems may result in bringing child misbehavior well within normal limits, with changes often maintained after the token system is discontinued. As a result, I strongly recommend the use of this method with all children 4 years of age and older who display oppositional or noncompliant behavior.

You should inform parents that many of them already employ an informal, less systematic reward program with their children. Parents often supplement their praise and attention for appropriate compliance with promises of special privileges, activities, allowances, or tangible rewards. The only additional procedure you introduce is a method of accounting that allows both the parent and the child to know whether the child has in fact earned the promised privilege. Furthermore, adopting a poker chip or point system also allows parents to reinforce child behaviors more quickly, resulting in greater control over child behavior. Such a system also allows parents to have some system of reward available at all times for use in managing the child.

Explain to parents that the home chip and point systems, or token economies, are very similar to the monetary system on which our society operates, except on a much smaller scale. Rather than using paper money and metal coins, the family will employ poker chips with young children (7 years and younger) while using points recorded in a notebook for older children. As in our large social economy, children in this system will be able to earn chips or points for "work" or compliance and exchange their earnings for a variety of rewards.

Experience with this program shows that children 3 years of age or younger do not respond as well, perhaps because they have not yet acquired the ability to comprehend symbolic reinforcers such as chips, points, or money. Further, their number concepts may not be adequately developed to allow appreciation for the units of payment to be used. For whatever reason, I discourage use of this program for children 3 years or younger. Parents can instead be taught to implement reinforcement programs that rely more on direct tangible rewards for the child, such as snacks, favorite drinks, stickers, or small toys to supplement parental use of attention and affection as rewards. For children 4–7 years of age, I recommend the use of a poker chip program, which permits the child to see and exchange tangible reinforcers (chips) as part of the program. For children 8 years and older, a point system by which the number of points earned or spent is recorded in a notebook is more useful and less offensive to the children. Clinical judgment should be used in deciding which reinforcement method to adopt. Some 8- or 9-year-olds may do better on a chip program than a point system. Parents can often suggest which program they believe would be more useful for their child.

Advantages of the Chip/Point System

The therapist should then elaborate for the parents the numerous advantages that accrue from use of a token reinforcement program. Briefly, these are as follows:

1. Token systems permit parents to *draw on more powerful rewards* for children in managing child behavior than mere social praise and attention will permit. Hence, greater and more rapid improvements in compliance can often be achieved beyond what social attention could accomplish.

2. Token systems are *highly convenient* reward systems. Chips or points can be taken anywhere, dispensed at anytime, and used to earn virtually any form of privilege or tangible incentive.

3. Token rewards are likely to *retain their value or effectiveness throughout the day* and across numerous situations. In contrast, children often become satiated quickly with food rewards, stickers, or other tangible reinforcers, resulting in a loss of motivating power as a behavior-change tool once the child is satiated. Because tokens can be exchanged for an almost limitless variety of rewards, their effectiveness as reinforcers is less likely to fluctuate with the children's level of satiation to a particular reward.

4. Token systems *permit a more organized, systematic, and fair approach* to managing children's behavior. The system makes it very clear what children earn for particular behaviors and what amount of points or chips is required for access to each privilege or reward. It also makes it equally clear to parents. This precludes the arbitrariness often seen in typical child management by parents where a child may be granted a reward or privilege on the spur of the moment because the parent is in a good mood rather than because the child has earned it. Similarly, it prevents parents from denying rewards that have been legitimately earned simply because the child misbehaved once during that day.

5. Token systems result in *increased parental attention to appropriate child behavior* and compliance. Because the parents must dispense the tokens, they must attend and respond more often to child behaviors they might otherwise have overlooked. The children also make parents more aware of their successes or accomplishments so as to earn the tokens.

6. Token systems teach a fundamental concept of society, and that is that privileges and rewards, as well as most of the things we desire in life, must be earned by the way we behave. This is the work ethic that parents naturally wish to instill in their children: The harder they work, and the more they apply themselves to handling responsibilities, the greater will be the rewards the children receive.

Establishing the Home Poker Chip Program

As noted above, the poker chip program is meant for children generally between the ages of 4 and 7 years. Parents can assist you in deciding whether poker chips or points will be the more effective token for their children. The guidelines for setting up the poker chip program are discussed here, while its modification into a point system is discussed in the next section. Parents should be given the handout for this session and then each step should be discussed in detail. The steps to setting up the chip program are as follows:

1. Decide what type of chip is to be used. I encourage parents to use the standard plastic poker chip, although some have used bingo chips, checkers, buttons, or other durable, small, yet convenient tokens. In using the colored poker chips, I have found it helpful to take one of each color (white, blue, and red) and to tape them to a small sheet of cardboard and display them in a convenient, visible location for easy reference by the child (say, the front of the kitchen refrigerator). On each chip, the parent should print the number of chips they represent. The white chip can be worth 1 chip, the blue one 5 chips, and the red one 10 chips. For 4- and 5-year-olds, this need not be done as each chip, regardless of color, represents only 1 chip.

2. The parents should take time to explain to the child the program that is about to be implemented. The parents can explain that they would like to provide the child with greater rewards for all of the work the child has been doing about the home. This often sets a positive tone in establishing the program rather than telling the child that, because of his/her misbehavior he/she is now going to have all privileges taken away and will have to earn them back again.

3. The parent and child should then construct a container that will serve as the bank for storing the chips earned by the child. Parents can make this fun by decorating a shoe box or large plastic jar with designs prepared by the child.

4. The parent should take time to sit down with the child and construct a list of privileges the child enjoys. Generally, children will suggest special or exceptional privileges that they do not ordinarily have available to them each day, such as going out to eat or to the movies, or buying toys. Parents can list these but should also include those privileges available each day, such as watching television, playing video games or a stereo, riding a bike, going to a friend's home, and so forth. The list should contain no less than 10 privileges; 15 is even better. Approximately one third of these should be short-term rewards that are available to the child every day and for which he/she will have to pay but a small number of chips. These are things like watching television, playing a video game, riding a bike, using roller blades, playing with special toys in the home, going to a neighborhood friend's home, having a special dessert after dinner, and so forth. Approximately one third of the privileges should be mid-term ones that will require several days of earnings to purchase. These can be things like staying up past bedtime, watching a special movie or television program not usually shown, spending the night at a friend's home, or helping the parents perform some desirable activity (baking, building things, etc.). At least one third of these should be highly desired long-term privileges such as buying things at the store, going to the movies or out to eat, renting a video movie to watch or a video game to play, taking a special trip, having a party with friends, and so forth. These will be more expensive privileges that the child will have to save for over several days to several weeks.

   Warning: Parents should not charge children for necessities, such as food, clothing, a bed, and the like.

5. Now the parent and child should cooperate in making a list of jobs, responsibilities, and other behaviors the parents wish to "target" to increase (sharing with a sibling, waiting one's turn to talk at the dinner table, etc.). These can include jobs such as making a bed, cleaning the bedroom, emptying trash cans, doing dishes, setting or clearing dishes for meals, doing homework, and so forth. In addition, certain responsibilities, such as dressing for school, dressing for bed, bathing, and the like, can be placed on the list if they have been problematic. The parent can also include social behaviors such as not swearing, not hitting, not lying, or not stealing. In order to reinforce a child for not doing something, parents must establish time periods after which they will pay the child for getting through without showing these undesirable behaviors. For instance, a child who often argues with a parent might be provided three chips for not arguing between breakfast and lunch, another three for not doing so between lunch and dinner, and a final three for the period from dinner to bedtime.

6. I also believe that parents should inform the child that "bonus chips" will be given for the attitude shown by the child during the performance of these jobs and behaviors. Such bonuses will not be paid every time the child does the job but are discretionary in that the parent can include them for a positive emotional demeanor by the child during performance of the task.

7. The parent should now take the list of jobs from item 5 above and decide how much is to be paid for each. For 4- and 5-year-olds, the range of chips can be between one and five; for older children a larger range of amounts can be used. In general, the more difficult and effortful the job or the more problematic the child has been previously in doing it, the more chips the parents will assign to that task.

8. Now the parent needs to decide how much to charge the child for each reward on the list. This can best be done by first adding up how many chips the child is likely to earn in an average day from doing the routine jobs listed in item 5 above. With this figure in mind, parents should assign enough chips to each privilege such that about two-thirds of the daily amount earned will be spent on those rewards the child will want each day (television, riding a bike, etc.). This leaves about one-third of the chips to be saved each day for spending on the mid- and long-term privileges on the list. These are just rough guidelines parents may wish to follow. Once the system is implemented, adjustments can be made to make the system more equitable. The more salient and expensive the privilege, the more chips the child will have to spend to earn it. Parents may wish to include money as a potential reward the child can purchase with the chips. If so, a limit is set as to how many chips can be cashed in each week for money to prevent the child from using chips to purchase only money. The money would be dispensed similar to an allowance.

9. The chip system is then implemented the week after these lists are constructed. I have found it helpful for young, prereading children to have their mothers construct separate lists for the rewards and jobs and then to draw pictures next to them that represent the job or reward. Parents may wish to skim through magazine ads to find pictures to cut out and paste next to the items on the lists.

Establishing the Home Point System

For children who are 8 years of age and older, points, rather than chips, are used as reinforcers. The parents take a notebook and organize it similar to a checkbook. Five columns in the notebook are created and are marked with date, item, deposit, withdrawal, and current balance, respectively. Then, whenever a child is to be rewarded for compliance, the parent enters the date, a brief notation in the "item" column as to the behavior performed, the amount of points earned in the "deposit" column, and then increases the balance reflecting the new deposit. When a child spends points on a reward or activity, the parent notes the type of reward in the "item" column, enters the amount spent under "withdrawal," and then deducts this amount from the balance. The child is never permitted to make entries in the notebook—only parents.

The list of privileges is constructed in the same way as described above for a chip program except, of course, that the privileges are appropriate to the older age of the child. In all likelihood, the list of jobs constructed will be somewhat larger than in the chip program because the child's greater abilities permit him/her to assist with more household chores than is the case with a younger child.

The number of points assigned to each privilege and each job on the lists is determined in much the same way as the point system. The harder the job, the more points paid for doing it. The more valuable the reward, the more points charged for it. The only difference between the chip and point systems is that larger amounts of points are used. I generally use a range of 20–200 points to be paid for the various jobs listed for the child. For instance, 15 points per 15 minutes of work can be used to determine how much to pay for protracted chores, such as homework, mowing the yard, and so forth. Similarly, a large range of points is assigned to the list of rewards and privileges.

Otherwise, the point system operates identically to the chip program. Both parents should utilize the system and both should award points as soon after the occurrence of compliance as possible. The lists of privileges and jobs should be reviewed periodically and changes made to keep them current with the desires of the children and parents.

Cautions in Starting the Program

Although the token programs are quite easy to implement and administer, there are certain precautions that parents should observe during the first few weeks of the program. These should be explained to the parents before the session is concluded. A major principle parents must follow during the first week is to use the chip program *only for rewarding good behavior*. Parents have a tendency to use the program to punish unacceptable behavior by taking back chips the child has earned unless they are forewarned not to do so during this first week. I have found that when parents use the program for penalizing children this first week, children often lose interest in the program before substantial motivation to participate in it can be generated. In subsequent weeks, you will explain how to use the program as a method of punishment, but this should not be permitted during the first week or so that the chip system is initially implemented. So, NO PENALTIES IN THE CHIP PROGRAM THIS WEEK!

Parents should also be cautioned that children are much more likely to want to participate in the chip system if parents go out of their way during the first week to give away more chips than they might normally do. The children should be rewarded for even the simplest of good behaviors to show them how easy it is to earn chips in the program and to enhance their desire to work within its guidelines. Parental stinginess with the chips during this week is very counterproductive to developing motivation of the children to cooperate with the procedures.

The parents must also be instructed that the chips are given only after a behavior or job has been performed, never before performance of the job upon which the chips are contingent. Some children attempt to barter with their parents or otherwise argue for an advance against future payments, especially if they wish to participate in some desirable activity now for which they do not yet have the requisite number of chips. The rule to follow is that if the child does not have the chips, he/she is not allowed access to the reward.

When the chips are administered, the parent should do so with a pleasant tone of voice, taking care to specify exactly what behavior is being rewarded and giving praise or appreciation to the child along with the chips. When chips are exchanged by the child for a reward, the child is to extract them from his/her bank and pay them to the parent. I discourage parents from making such withdrawals, as I believe the actual motoric act of both withdrawing and depositing the chips in the bank enhances the program's effectiveness.

With children who are likely to steal, parents should be certain that the container of chips to be earned is kept out of reach of the children so that pilfering is discouraged. The child is only permitted to touch those chips in his/her own bank.

If both parents are in the home, both should be strongly encouraged to utilize the chips as rewards. There is a tendency for mothers to play the predominant role in this program. Although this may at times be justified by one parent's spending greater amounts of time with the child, the other parent should be encouraged to award chips during the time he/she is with the child. This enhances consistency of child management procedures between the parents.

The chips can be used to reward virtually any type of appropriate child behavior, even if it is not on the list. Parents should be reminded of this, as some are likely to follow the guidelines of the program quite rigidly, thereby missing opportunities to reinforce compliance. Parents can also begin using the chips to reward children for independent play during times when the parent is busy. The method of shaping discussed in Step 3 can be readily reinforced with chips in addition to attention. The chips are to be dispensed immediately upon the occurrence of child compliance. The greater the delay in dispensing the chips, the less control the program will exert over child compliance.

Every few weeks, parents should review the list of rewards with the child to see if new ones should be added, or others dropped from the list because they are never requested by the child. In addition, new jobs and responsibilities can be added to the list as parent and child see fit.

I have found it useful for parents to stop their activities periodically throughout the day, say every 20–30 minutes, in order to monitor their child's activities to determine if a reward is appropriate at that time. Some parents choose to set the alarm on their kitchen cooking timer to assist in reminding them of this monitoring. Others can use wrist watches that permit programming of such alarms. In a few cases, I have suggested that parents place small stickers, such as "smiley face" stickers, throughout the home in places where they commonly look. These stickers serve as reminders to observe and reinforce child behaviors whenever the parent sees a sticker. Such places as the faces of clocks, mirrors, the handle of the telephone, and the control panel of the television set can be excellent places to put such sticker cues to prompt monitoring and reinforcement of the child.

Parents must be patient with this program. Although many children show changes in compliance during the first day the system is implemented, others take several days to a week before the program is sufficiently motivating to increase child compliance. A few oppositional children may even refuse to participate in the procedure, believing that if they stall and withhold participation the parent will give up using the procedure. In such cases, parents are told that the program is to stay in effect regardless of the children's initial reaction to it. The children simply do not get access to the rewards on the list unless they have earned the chips to do so. Some of these children may spend a few days without any privileges or rewards until this principle is fully appreciated. At this point, the children grudgingly begin to cooperate. This is a rare reaction, however, as the vast majority of children find the program to be quite a positive one.

Common Parental Reactions

Many parents wish to know if siblings, babysitters, or relatives can use the chip or point systems with the children. I generally permit siblings to reward or take away tokens from a child only if they are in their late teenage years and can be trusted by the parents to use the program fairly and in accord with the guidelines described above. The same applies to babysitters. If the same babysitter is commonly used and the sitter is a late teenager or young adult, then they may use the token system with the child. Again, parental judgment must be exercised to ensure that the system is used fairly with the children. I typically discourage relatives from using the token systems unless they are in frequent contact with the children and have major caregiving responsibilities for them, such as serving as babysitters while the mother or father of the child is working.

Many parents believe that token systems constitute bribery of the child. This reflects a misunderstanding of the concept of bribery. Bribery is the offer of an incentive for performance of an illicit, immoral, or illegal act by another person. Clearly, this is not the case within this token system. The system is very similar to the parents being paid for working outside the home and is simply a fair wage for a fair day's work by the child. Usually, the complaint of bribery actually relates to parental concerns that the child is being rewarded for doing things that other children are not given rewards for performing. As noted earlier, you may have to explain the notion of a behavioral handicap in the child with ADHD whereby the token system serves as a prosthetic device permitting the child to overcome his/her handicap. Without the device, the child remains handicapped. With it, the child may perform activities similar to those that normal children do without the prosthetic device. Whether or not this explanation is given, parents should be told that normal children *are* rewarded for behaving well; they are just not rewarded so systematically. Normal children are often provided with privileges, treats, or other rewards but the fact that they are given for good behavior is often not made explicit or even contingent upon the imme-diately preceding occurrence of good behavior. Nonetheless, let the normal child drift into noncompliant or defiant behavior and such privileges are often quickly withdrawn, albeit temporarily, until better behavior is evident.

Some parents believe the token system will be too time consuming for them. Here you may have to confront the parents as to how motivated they are to help in the behavioral recovery of their child. Parents can be reassured that although the program takes a little more time during its initial few weeks of usage, it will eventually become a habit for the parents and of little inconvenience if they will only stay with the program for a while.

Parents often wish to know if other siblings should be placed on the program. This must be a decision made on the basis of each family's circumstances. The parents can discuss it with the siblings to get their opinion or may simply decide that all children in the family will be on chip or point systems. Certainly, the greater the number of children in a family, the more burdensome the system becomes for the parents. Often, siblings ask to be placed on a similar program because they see how participation in it leads to a clear knowledge of what is required to earn privileges.

A few parents ask when they can stop the procedure and how to do so. It is interesting that such parents wish to discuss stopping treatment even before it is implemented. I generally stipulate that the program must remain in effect for 2 months (until the 1-month booster session) as a minimum period. If need be, a session with the family can be held at that time to discuss the gradual phasing out of the program. However, many families will find that the program dies a natural death, gradually being phased out without any systematic effort to do so. Parents tend to become inconsistent with the method after several months, espe-cially if the child has been behaving quite well. If parents wish to remove the program for-mally, I suggest that the child be told that the token system will be removed for 1 or 2 days to see how well the child behaves without it. The child will still have his/her rewards and privileges, but they will be granted based on whether or not the work has been done or the child has been compliant with most requests. If the child is able to sustain his/her compli-ance during this trial period, then the parents can continue to extend the trial period indefi-nitely. If problems arise, the child can be returned to the program quite quickly.

Homework

The parents should continue the special playtime periods with the child as well as work-ing on rewarding the child for compliance and for playing independently of the parents (i.e., not interrupting them when they are busy) as was taught in Step 3. The major as-signment for this session is to implement the token system. If it was not done so in the session itself, parents are to construct the lists of responsibilities and privileges within a day or so after the session and to implement the system. They are to bring these lists to the next session for review by the therapist. If the child is on a point system, his/her "bank" book is to be brought to this session.

Time Out! and Other Disciplinary Methods

Goals

1. To introduce the use of fines into the home token system as punishment for non-compliance and unacceptable social conduct.
2. To train parents in the use of an effective time out (isolation) method as punishment for selected child misbehavior.

Materials Required

- Parent Handout for Step 5
    Time Out!

Step Outline

- Review homework
    Make adjustments to the home token system
- Discuss the use of the token system for penalties (response cost procedure)
- Prepare parents for importance of the session
    It is the most difficult week of the program
    It requires the utmost consistency
- Distribute the parent handout
- Thoroughly review all steps of the procedure
    How to use time out for noncompliance
    Where the time out chair should be located
    How long the child should remain in the chair
    What to do if the child leaves the chair without permission

Ploys the child may use to avoid time out
How to manage physical resistance by the child

- Review restrictions to using time out this week
- Discuss parent reactions to the procedure
- Model the procedure

Homework

- Implement behavioral penalties
- Use time out for only one or two noncompliant behaviors
- Record use of all time outs
- Continue previously taught methods

This session begins with a review of the lists from the token system implemented during the previous week. Time is taken to troubleshoot any problems that may have arisen, make adjustments to the amounts being awarded or charged for various items on the list, deal with any questions the parents and children may have about continued used of the program, and encourage the parents in its continued use. Many parents will report dramatic changes in child behavior as a result of these token systems. Even if parents believe there are no further behavioral problems with the child, they should still be taught the use of penalties and the time out procedure. There is certainly an initial honeymoon period with the token system (usually 3–4 weeks), in my experience, and the parents must be prepared for the occasional return of some noncompliant behavior even if the child is now behaving normally.

Implementing a Response Cost Procedure

The token system lends itself for use as a form of punishment for unacceptable behavior or noncompliance that is as effective as the reward program is for compliant behavior. The parent merely removes a certain number of chips or points as a penalty for the child not doing a chore or failing to follow a command or rule. Generally, the amount deducted is the same amount that would have been awarded had the child performed the chore. For instance, if a child normally receives five chips for making his/her bed upon request, then if the child fails to do so he/she must pay the parent five chips from his/her bank. This is in addition to the opportunity the child has just missed to earn five more chips.

Parents may now wish to develop a short list of undesirable social behaviors performed by the child. This list will consist of those frequently occurring unacceptable behaviors that will now be fined via tokens should they be displayed by the child. Such behaviors as aggression, lying, stealing, arguing, swearing, or other violations of household rules may be placed on this list. The more severe the misbehavior, the greater the penalty assigned.

Parents must be cautioned about a problem that often arises in using tokens in a response cost or penalty procedure such as this. I call it the "punishment spiral." This occurs when a parent fines a child for misbehavior and the child responds with a tantrum, swearing, or destructiveness. These reactions are then fined because they, too, are unacceptable. This further provokes the child's negative reaction and the child escalates to further verbal abuse of the parent or destructiveness, which then leads to further fines under the response cost program, and so on. The net effect is a spiraling of parental punishment entwined with escalating negative reactions by the child to a point where the child has been fined more points than he/she can ever hope to earn and therefore loses all motivation for the program. This dilemma can be managed by the parent by following this rule: A child is fined once through the point system and then if a negative reaction ensues the child is sent to time out (as described below).

Preparing the Parents for Using Time Out

It is a major purpose of this session to assist the family in developing a more effective style of disciplining the child for noncompliance and other inappropriate behaviors. In doing so, it is essential that you prepare the family for several things that will take place during the coming homework assignment. First, the parents should be prepared for the fact that this will probably be the most difficult week of the program for them. In many cases when the time out procedure is implemented, children may throw temper tantrums lasting as long as an hour or more, which may prove quite aversive or distressing to the parents. During these tantrums, the parents may feel as if they should give in to their child in order to terminate this unpleasant behavior and the harm the parents believe this penalty is causing the child. Although this parental response would certainly be effective at ceasing such crying or reducing the child's disruptiveness, it would merely serve to reinforce the future occurrence of such behavior. Thus, once the time out procedure has been instituted, the parents must see it to its final conclusion without acquiescing to the child's tantrums. Parents should be warned to expect a high rate of negative child reactions when time out is first implemented and that this, in fact, reflects that the method will probably eventually prove effective with that child.

A second factor for which the parents must be prepared is to use discipline consistently for the child's noncompliance, even if it may inconvenience them to do so. Up to this point, the parents have probably been quite inconsistent in the manner in which they have handled the child's misbehavior. Inconsistency is often found even between parents in that one employs a more strict technique than the other, who may in fact become less strict to compensate for this. Parental inconsistency greatly weakens the effectiveness of this procedure and makes it harder to implement successfully on subsequent occasions.

Third, parents should reduce special family activities to a minimum during the coming week so that parents may devote more time to seeing that this time out method is correctly employed. If special activities cannot be rescheduled (e.g., weddings, visits by out-of-state relatives, etc.), then you should postpone teaching the procedure until after the special activities have been completed.

Instructing Parents in the Time Out Procedure

This is one of the most effective methods in this program but must be taught with great care and implemented by the parents in close accord with the explanation you will provide. Give the parents the handout and allow adequate time for them to read it.

Parents are taught that from this point forward, when the parents give a command to the child, they should be prepared to back it up with consequences for noncompliance. If they are not willing to do so, then the command should not be issued. The consequences are to be implemented immediately and commands are not to be repeated to the child.

When a command is given, the parent should view the sequence of procedures to be followed as occurring in three stages. I often use the analogy of a stoplight to describe these three stages. The first stage involves the parent giving the command in a neutral but businesslike tone of voice. The command is not to be phrased as a question or favor but as an imperative. The parent should follow all of the guidelines reviewed in Step 3 for giving effective commands. Once the command is issued, the parent counts backward from 5 to 1 out loud to permit 5 seconds or so to elapse and to signal clearly to the child that a very short interval exists in which to initiate compliance. After a few weeks, I encourage parents to cease using countdowns like this out loud so as to avoid teaching the child to obey only those commands followed by countdowns; at this time, parents simply count to themselves for 5 seconds. Issuing the first command is the green light of the traffic signal—everything is still "go" between the parent and child in that no unpleasant or noncompliant behaviors have yet occurred.

After the 5-second countdown has elapsed, if the child has not yet begun to comply, the parent then issues a warning. This is the yellow warning light of a traffic signal, to follow our analogy further. Like the traffic signal, the parent's warning is to be distinct from the first command. The parent is instructed to make direct eye contact, to raise his/her voice to a louder level (not yelling), to adopt a firmer posture and stance, to point a finger at the child, and to present the child with the warning, "If you don't do as I say, then you are going to sit in that chair!" The parent points directly to the vicinity where the time out chair is situated. The entire display by the parent should be so constructed as to convey unequivocally to the child that the parent means what he/she is threatening and will not hesitate to place the child in the chair.

After the warning, the parent again counts down from 5 to 1 to permit another 5 seconds to elapse. If the child has not begun to comply within this time interval, the parent proclaims to the child, "You did not do as I said; now you are going to the chair!" The parent then takes the child firmly by the upper arm or wrist and escorts the child quickly to the time out chair, placing the child firmly in the seat. The parent then states, firmly and loudly, "You stay there until I say you can get up!" This step clearly constitutes the red light in the analogy.

At this point, no more than 15 seconds have elapsed since the first command was given. As a result, parents find they are not emotionally out of control as they might have been had they repeated their commands or warnings multiple times without gaining compliance. The punishment is therefore implemented at a time when the parent is most capable of pursuing it in a systematic and businesslike fashion. The therapist should decide how loud, firm, and theatrical the parents' display of the warning is to be for the level of severity of the child's behavioral disorder. Mildly disordered children may not require or deserve as loud a warning or intense a parental display over noncompliance as more severely disordered children.

The child is to be taken immediately to the chair once the 5-second count has occurred. Some children may promise to comply at this point, having seen the parent reaching for them to implement the time out. However, it is too late for that, and the parents are to implement the time out method despite the child's attempt at compliance. The time for compliance is now over and the punishment cannot be avoided. Other children will try to resist the time out by complaining, threatening, or throwing a tantrum. The parent is to escort the child, physically if necessary, to the chair regardless of the child's reaction. In short, nothing the child can do will prevent the punishment from being implemented once the 5-second compliance interval has elapsed.

Where Should the Chair Be Located?

As the parent handout suggests, there are several appropriate places for the time out chair. The chair should not be located in a closet, a bathroom, or the child's bedroom. It should be placed in a spot that is convenient for the parent to supervise while the parent continues his/her housework. A corner of a foyer, the dining room, the kitchen, or the middle of a hallway are commonly used places. The chair should be a straight-backed dinette-style chair such as that used in a kitchen dinette set, and it should be placed a sufficient distance from the wall such that the child cannot kick the wall without leaving the chair. There should be nothing within easy reach of the child with which he/she can play. The chair should be left out, visible to the child throughout the day, for at least 2 weeks, as it will serve as a good reminder of what consequence will occur for noncompliance.

How Long Should the Child Remain in Time Out?

There are numerous variations of time out reinforcement, each with its own recommended length of time. Many employ a standard time period, regardless of the age of the child.

However, this fails to respect the fact that a child's perception of time varies with his/her developmental level. Young children clearly require less time out before they experience the isolation as unpleasant, as compared to older children who may require a longer interval to have the same subjective impression of unpleasantness. In the present method, a length of time is assigned based on the age of the child. There are essentially three conditions that must be met *in sequence* by the child before the time out is terminated.

1. The child must serve a "minimum sentence" as punishment for the infraction. This is to be 1–2 minutes per year of the child's age. A 4-year-old would serve a minimum of 4 minutes in time out, for instance.

2. Once the minimum sentence has elapsed, the child must be quiet for a few moments. The child need not be quiet during the minimum sentence interval, but once that has elapsed, the child must be quiet before the parent will approach the chair. The child may be told this on the first occasion time out is used in this program. The parent would say, "I am not coming back to the chair until you are quiet." This should not be repeated. The child must be quiet for about 30 seconds to meet this second condition. When time out is first used, many children will continue to be vocally disruptive after the minimum sentence has elapsed, and may continue this behavior for several minutes to several hours (in rare cases). If so, the child is to remain in time out until he/she has become quiet, even if it initially extends the time out episode to 1–2 hours. Experience has shown that after this initial confrontation over the first time out, the length of time children require in time out diminishes greatly as they learn that becoming quiet quickly shortens the time out interval.

3. Finally, the child must consent to do the original directive. For instance, if the child failed to pick up toys and this resulted in being sent to the time out chair, then the child must agree to pick up the toys. If the behavior that resulted in time out cannot be corrected (e.g., the child hit someone or swore at a parent), then the child must agree not to display that behavior again. In other words, the child promises not to repeat that behavior. In the future, should the child do so, he/she would be immediately taken to the time out chair without a command or warning being given. If the child should refuse to perform the requested task or refuse to make the promise not to repeat the behavior, then the child is told, "All right, then you stay there until I say you can get up!". At this point, the three conditions are to be repeated: The child serves another minimum sentence, must be quiet for a few moments, and must then consent to do what he/she was told. This sequence repeats itself until the child agrees to do what he/she was asked or promises not to display the misbehavior again, depending on the reason time out was implemented.

While the child is in the chair, there is to be no discussion or argument with the child. The parent is to return to housework or other activity, although keeping an eye out for the child's behavior while in the chair. Siblings and the other spouse are not to speak with the child.

Once the child has done what was asked, then the parent is to indicate in a neutral tone of voice that he/she likes it when the child listens to the parent. No tokens are to be given at this point for compliance nor is the parent to make any apology, as some parents tend to do, for having had to punish the child. The parent should then monitor the child's behavior for the next occurrence of important appropriate behavior and reinforce the child for that positive behavior. This is done to keep an appropriate balance between positive reinforcement and punishment within this program as well as to show the child that the parent does not dislike him/her but was punishing the child for misbehavior.

There are certain instances in which this entire sequence of events would not be followed (i.e., command, warning, then time out). These instances are either when a previously stated household rule has been violated or when the parent is assigning a chore that requires an extended time period to accomplish. In the first case, the child may have violated a clearly understood rule of the household, such as no hitting, no stealing, no taking food from the kitchen without permission, no playing with Dad's power tools, and so forth. In such a case, the child would be sent to time out immediately without the rule being repeated or a warning given. I often direct parents to post a list of commonly violated household rules in a visible location (refrigerator door) when starting this program and to tell the child that violation of those rules leads to immediate placement in the time out chair without warning. In the second case, where the chore given to the child requires extended time to accomplish (clean your room, do your homework, etc.), the parent is to give both the command and warning at the same time. For example, the child is told to clean his/her bedroom, is given 15 minutes to do so, and then is warned that if the room is not clean by then, he/she will go to time out. This can all be stated by the parent when the initial request is made. The parent should be told to set the time interval on a kitchen timer such that both parent and child will know when the time has expired, avoiding arguments over whether the time has in fact elapsed.

What If the Child Leaves the Chair without Permission?

You should review the options that parents have for ensuring that a child remains in the chair until the parent states that time out is over. The option that I frequently employ is to send the child to his/her bedroom to serve the time out period. The child is to sit on the bed during this period. The door may be left open, but if the child attempts to leave the room, it will be closed and locked until the three conditions discussed above for release from time out have occurred. Other options will be discussed, but they are believed to be less effective.

When the child first leaves the chair without permission, the parent is to provide a warning. This warning is provided only once, on the first occasion the child leaves the chair, and is never repeated during subsequent uses of time out. The parent returns the child to the chair and states, "If you get out of that chair again, I am going to send you to your bed!" This is said quite loudly as the parent points a finger at the child, again adopting a firm stance and posture. Thereafter, should the child ever leave the chair again without permission, the parent sends the child to his/her bedroom and places the child on the bed. The child is then told to stay there until the parent has indicated that the child can leave the room. If the bedroom is used for this purpose, it should be stripped of all major toys or other play activities (e.g., television, video games, stereos, etc.) until the child's behavior has improved to a point where time out is not being used very often.

A few parents may not wish to isolate their child to a bedroom when the child leaves time out. There are several alternatives for the parents who wish not to use the isolation method. The parent may deduct a certain number of tokens from the child's bank account for every infraction of time out, but there are limits to this procedure. A second alternative is to threaten the child with removal of some later privilege (watching television, going to a friend's house later that day, etc.) should the child leave time out prematurely. This may work well for older children, provided the privilege to be removed is an especially salient one for the child. Finally, the child's time out interval can be extended an additional 5 minutes for every time he/she leaves the chair. I do not favor this option, partially because there is a limit to this, of course, before the interval becomes ridiculously long due to numerous infractions of the time out procedure. Also, this may lead to a game of "cat and mouse," which the child may find entertaining and which certainly results in his/her not being isolated from the family or from parental attention.

Ploys Some Children Use to Avoid/Escape Time Out

There are several common ploys that children have used in attempting to escape or avoid the use of the time out procedure by their parents. Two were already noted above, these being the children's promising to do a task once they see their parents are serious about taking them to the time out chair, and the other being children's refusal to go to time out. In either case, the parental response is the same—the children are taken to time out immediately, using slight physical force if need be to achieve that end. However, once in the chair (or bedroom), these children often make further efforts at escape before the time out interval has been satisfactorily served. Listed below are a few common ploys and how they should be managed:

1. *The child asks to go to the bathroom.* Virtually all of the children whom I have treated have been fully capable of controlling their bowel and bladder functions for the short interval of time they are in time out. As a result, parents should be instructed that no child is to be permitted to leave time out to use the bathroom. They may do so once the three conditions for terminating time out have been met, as described above. Many children threaten that they will wet themselves if not permitted to use the bathroom, but in the 20 years I have used this program, only two children have done so and in both cases it was obviously an intentional display of opposition and defiance to the parents. In both cases, the children remained in time out until the specified conditions were met. They then

had to clean up the area and change their clothing once they had complied with the initial command. If children are permitted to leave the time out area prematurely to use the bathroom, common sense dictates that they will employ this tactic frequently thereafter whenever sent to time out and will likely use the time in the bathroom for play. No doubt it will also be difficult to get them to return to the time out area once so released from it.

2. *The child claims he/she will not love that parent anymore.* Whereas most parents see this statement as the temporary, emotionally laden, and manipulative comment that it is, a few are truly upset that their children might say such things. Such parents are apparently so insecure in their relationship with the child that they may capitulate and release the child from time out when such a statement is made. Other parents may not go to that extreme of appeasement but may nonetheless experience great guilt and anxiety while the child is uttering such phrases of hatred against the parent during the time out interval. You must prepare the parents for such remarks, discuss in advance how they might feel about hearing them, and then direct them not to react outwardly to them in any way while the child is in time out. Reassuring the child of parental affection only provides attention to the child during time out and fosters further arguments and tirades against the parents in future episodes of time out.

3. *The child attempts to move the chair or tip it over.* As noted above, such activities are construed as having left the chair without permission and should be managed by the use of an initial warning or threat of sending the child to the bedroom if such behavior persists. In cases where parents have chosen not to use the bedroom isolation procedure, the alternative they have selected would be used to respond to these instances of rocking, moving, or tipping over the time out chair.

4. *The child threatens he/she will get sick and may vomit.* Several children treated in our clinic each year use the ploy of illness to gain escape from time out. Some state that they have a sore throat (no doubt from all their tantruming), while others complain of headaches or stomachaches. Parents should be taught that the child is merely going through the hierarchy of manipulative behaviors that he/she has found successful on previous occasions to see if they will work in this instance. Parents should ignore such statements, unless there is objective evidence of illness prior to having sent the child to time out (e.g., child has had a cold or flu that day). Once the child discovers that such complaints no longer elicit parental sympathy and attention, they will not be used in subsequent situations when time out is implemented. However, if attended to by a guilt-ridden parent, they would no doubt be used again by the child in future episodes of time out. I have known of one child who actually threatened to vomit if not released from time out. This was a mildly retarded, conduct-problem child who had used such a strategy at school successfully to gain teacher attention and avoid punishment. The parents were instructed to ignore such a threat, and the child actually made good on the warn-

ing by sticking his finger down his throat and vomiting. The parents were told to require the child to remain in the time out chair until the three conditions above were met, at which point not only did he have to comply with the initial command but he was also made to clean up the mess created in the time out area. Obviously, such reactions from children to time out are extremely rare, but all parents should be instructed in how to manage them should theirs prove to be that rare child.

5. *The child complains of being tired or hungry.* Generally, these complaints arise when time out is implemented at bedtime (usually for failing to prepare for bed when asked) or at mealtimes. Parents are to be told that the child is to be sent to time out, even if it means keeping the child up past bedtime to do so. A few parents wonder if this isn't actually reinforcing to the child because he/she gets to stay up past bedtime. My experience has been that few children desire to stay up past bedtime to sit in a chair in a dull corner of the house alone while others are in the family room watching television. Usually, children wish to stay up past bedtime to remain in the presence of the family, to play, or to continue watching television. Thus, the children will not enjoy the time out and are not likely to behave in such a way at bedtime as to get sent to time out again. However, the therapist should note to the parents that what makes time out effective is what the children are missing while being in isolation. Because the children are missing little at bedtime other than sleep, the "minimum sentence" of time out at bedtime may have to be slightly longer (2 minutes per year of age) to make it effective as punishment.

For children who complain of hunger or are missing a family meal while in time out, parents are told that the children are simply to miss that meal but will be allowed to eat again when the next meal is scheduled. Parents are not to go out of their way to save the children's meal for them or to prepare a special meal once the time out episode has ended. If such were to happen, it is highly likely that time out during mealtimes would prove an inadequate form of punishment as the children are missing little if anything during the time out interval. If the child should end the time out interval while the family is still completing a meal, he/she is permitted to return to the table to eat, but gets no additional time for eating when the rest of the family finishes dinner. At that point, the child's plate would be removed even if he/she had not yet finished the meal. In short, when children are sent to time out, they miss those activities occurring in the family during that time, and these are not to be made up later by the parents.

6. *The child refuses to leave time out.* On occasion, a child may refuse to leave the time out chair once the parent grants permission. Such an instance is a clear bid by the child to continue to control the parent–child interaction. In such cases, the parent is to tell the child that, because the child did not do what he/she was told (leave the chair), the child must sit there again until the parent says it is time to leave. In

this instance, the parent assigns another minimum sentence, then awaits the child's becoming quiet, and then approaches the child to see if he/she agrees to do what he/she was told.

Using Time Out with Physically Aggressive Children

A few children treated each year in our clinic, although young in age and small of size, threaten their parents with violence should the parent try to implement time out with them. Here, careful clinical judgment is required. Some children with a history of violence against others may well be sufficiently dangerous, even to their parents, that residential treatment of such children may be required initially to gain control over such behavioral patterns. However, other children are not so dangerous but still cause their parents some fear, especially their mothers, when they make such threats or in fact adopt a pose that is physically threatening to the parent when time out is to be initiated. In my experience, these have always been threats against the mother, not the father. Should the mother sufficiently fear such a response, I have recommended that the mother use time out only for a behavior problem that occurs when the father is typically at home. Time out is not to be used for any other occasions. In such cases, the child will often cooperate with time out, fearing that the father will join the interaction if need be to ensure that time out is implemented. When such children cooperate with time out imposed by the mother, the mother is told to tell the child that the time out period will be reduced somewhat because of the child's cooperation. After several weeks of using the procedure while the father is in the home, the mother is instructed to try it when the father is absent from the home. Presumably, the previous few weeks of cooperation from the child with the time out method will generalize to these instances of father absence. Where this fails, consideration should be given to inpatient treatment of this rare, assaultive child.

Common Parental Reactions to the Procedure

Most parents will be more than willing to implement these procedures with the child during subsequent weeks. Some parents, however, have concerns about the program or reservations about using it. One common parental reaction is that the parents have tried this method of time out before but that it has not worked for them. The therapist can explain that it is quite likely that the earlier version of time out was probably flawed in several respects. First, it is likely that the parents did not implement the program until they were quite angry and frustrated with the child and had repeated their commands many times in order to get the child to comply. This is hardly effective, as time out was used infrequently, not immediately upon the occurrence of the noncompliance, and when the parent was most likely to use an excessive time out period out of anger.

Second, most parents have used time out in a manner that has allowed control of the interval to remain in the hands of the child. That is, they have told the child to go to his/her room and stay there until he/she was ready to come out and behave properly. This obviously leaves the determination of when to end time out to the child.

A third mistake is that parents have often used a standard time out interval, say 5 minutes, for every episode of child misbehavior, regardless of the severity of the infraction or the age of the child. The problem here is that for older children the time out period is too short to be aversive and hence will be ineffective. Furthermore, the time out procedure should be adjusted to fit the severity of the rule violation. This is why this program recommends a range of 1–2 minutes for each year of the child's age. Modest rule infractions receive the smaller amount of time out, while serious infractions receive the larger amount.

Finally, it is likely that most parents did not use time out consistently for past misbehavior, thus detracting from its effectiveness. Often the parents used time out only when they were emotionally upset and not for the same rule infraction at other times when they were not so upset. Similarly, the parents may have allowed the child to barter his/her way out of time out by agreeing to comply with the command once it was clear that the parent was about to take the child to a time out location. The present program dictates that once the parent starts to implement time out, it is to be carried through no matter what the child promises to do for the parent at that moment.

Many parents inquire as to how they should use the procedure if there are visitors in the home. Their concern here appears to be one of fear of embarrassing the child or themselves. The parents should be told to implement the procedure regardless of the visitors. While apologies may have to be made to the visitors for doing so, this should not preclude the use of the time out procedure. Failure to implement time out in such cases would teach the child that occasions when visitors are in the home are ones in which the child can misbehave with immunity. If the visitors are neighborhood friends of the child, they should be asked to leave once time out has had to be implemented.

Restrictions on Using Time Out during the First Week

If parents were initially to use the time out procedure for all instances of noncompliance, many behavior disorderd children would spend the majority of their day in the chair in a corner. To avoid this excessive disciplining of the child, parents are told that they may use time out for only one or two noncompliant behaviors during the coming week, and these are to be ones occurring only in the home, not in public. I also suggest that the parents wait for a week before tackling bedtime problems. This allows the child to become accustomed to the time out procedure and for the possibility that its effects will generalize to commands given at bedtime, such that parents may not actually have to use the procedure at bedtime. They may wish to choose particular commands that are problematic for the child, such as picking up toys, getting dressed for school, or doing homework. Others will choose household rules that are frequently violated, such as hitting, swearing, or lying. In either case, only two commands or rules are to be chosen for use with the time out method.

The restriction against using the method in public places for the time being is founded on the belief that the time out procedure requires slight modification to be effective in public places. Parents also must be prepared for possible reactions from others who witness their use of time out with a child. In addition, by introducing the procedure at home for several weeks, it is possible that improvement in the home will be generalized to commands given in public places. In other words, once the children realize the parents "mean business" and have used the time out method when it was threatened, they may learn not to disobey commands or warnings issued in public places, where its use will also be threatened.

Parents should also be told that should they encounter problems with the procedure, they should call you immediately. Clinicians using this program should routinely give parents their home and work telephone numbers for use during this week should problems arise. It is extremely rare that any parents will call, but the security of knowing the therapist is readily available and the feelings this conveys to the parents of the importance of the procedures are quite therapeutic.

Parents will often ask what they should do to manage misbehaviors that are not to be the object of time out this week. They should be reminded of the availability of the response cost method (fining tokens for misbehavior), which can be used with any behavior problem. In some instances, parents may choose to use both methods of punishment for especially serious rule infractions. In this case, the child would be fined tokens from his/her bank account as well as sent to the time out chair for a longer-than-usual minimum sentence.

Modeling the Procedure

Throughout the discussion of the procedure, you can demonstrate the methods, with one of the parents pretending to be a child for the sake of modeling the sequence of events in a group setting. If an individual family is undergoing the training and the child is present, you may role play the method with the child, being certain to explain to the child that it is only pretend for now and that he/she will not be required to stay in time out. The parent is then to role play the method, with you serving as the pretend child. Forehand and McMahon (1981) suggest that the parent never serve as the child during role play in front of the child, as it may teach the child that the parent can be punished or placed in time out.

The parent and child can then be placed in a playroom together and the parent required to issue a variety of commands to the child until one is disobeyed. At this point the parent implements time out so that you can evaluate how well it is being used by the parent. Older children who have heard you explain the method usually will not violate parental commands in the playroom, as they realize what the consequences will be. In such cases, role playing the procedure will have to suffice. Role playing is also the mode of parental practice when this procedure is taught as part of a group parent training class. At first, you should choose a parent to serve as the pretend child for the role-play demonstration. Then the parents pair off and practice with other parents, taking turns in practicing the parental role in the procedure under your supervision.

Homework

Parents will of course continue to use the previously taught procedures. I often find at this step that parents begin to discontinue the special playtimes. They should be encouraged to keep these activities going, particularly this week, as they will serve to offset the deleterious effects of the punishment program on the parent–child relationship.

Besides implementing the time out procedure, parents are to record in a diary every instance when time out was employed, what the child did to receive time out, and how well the parents felt the procedure was implemented. Parents should also record the length of each time out episode. Before leaving the session, parents are to stipulate to the therapist the two noncompliant behaviors with which they will employ time out this week, as well as the location in the home where the time out is to be served.

Extending Time Out to Other Misbehavior

Goals

1. To troubleshoot and resolve problems parents are encountering in using the time out method with the child.

2. Where appropriate, to extend the use of the time out method to other commands or rules that elicit noncompliance.

Step Outline

- Review homework records on time out
- Reassess child disruptive behavior using rating scales
- Select two or more additional noncompliant behaviors for use with time out

Homework

- Continue using and recording time out method

The session begins with the usual review of parent homework records and discussion of problems the parents may have had in implementing the time out method. The majority of this session is spent in reviewing the instances in which time out was used, how the parents felt about it, problems that may have been encountered in its implementation, and any minor adjustments that may have to be made to the parents' use of the procedures. No new material is introduced in this session. For some families, the session will be brief, as they have been successfully using the procedure since the

Assigning the child an activity to perform

Monitoring, attending to, and rewarding compliance in the public place

- Review types of public places in which methods can be used

  Stores

  Restaurants

  During car travel

  While visiting others

  Church

- Review how to use methods for transitions between major activities

- Review and discuss parental reactions to methods

Homework

- Make two bogus shopping trips for practice

- Record information concerning these trips

- Contact child's teachers for updated report of child's school conduct

Reassessment of Child Disruptive Behavior

After reviewing the homework and resolving any minor problems the parents may still be having in their use of the time out procedure, have parents complete another set of the HSQ and DBDRS-PF rating scales so as to evaluate improvement in the child's disruptive behavior from the training program. Typically, the sessions dealing with the home token system and time out are the two most effective in this program and result in significant improvements in child compliance and disruptive behavior.

Anticipating Problems

Introduce the new material for this session by discussing the kinds of problems the parents are facing in managing their child in public. After a detailed review of these problems, introduce the notion that most parents do not think ahead about the kinds of problems they may face with a child in public places. Instead, many parents enter public places such as stores without a thought as to how they will cope with a behavior problem from the child should it arise. Only when the noncompliance or behavior problem occurs does the parent begin to think about how to deal with it. This is probably the worst time to begin planning a strategy for managing the problem, as the child will certainly be disruptive, the parent is likely to be angry, and the parent is likely to be anxious because of others watching this scene. All of these factors will detract from developing a reasonable and effective method of dealing with the problem.

As a result, anticipating behavioral problems is a key concept in learning to manage children effectively, both in public places and across transitions in major daily activities. I will deal with public places first, then discuss using the methods for activity transitions. Many parents have sufficient experience to know what types of public places are likely to evoke noncompliant behaviors and what type of behavioral problem is likely to arise. If parents would therefore take a few moments before entering such places in order to develop a plan to use should noncompliance occur and to make this plan clear to the child, much child misbehavior in public places could be avoided. In those cases where problems were not avoided, at least the parent would have established a quick and effective reaction to managing the misbehavior long before it attracts the attention of others in that setting.

Emphasis needs to be given to two concepts: (1) anticipation, or planning, in coping with the misbehavior of children in public places; and (2) the use of planned activities to be assigned to children to keep them busy and engaged in prosocial behavior during the public outing.

Distributing and Reviewing the Parent Handout

The handout for this session is brief, quite clear, and easily implemented by most parents. You should review it with parents step by step, in as much detail and with as many examples as necessary to illustrate the procedure. Essentially, the methods are no different than those previously taught but include some minor modifications allowing for the fact that no time out chair is readily available in public places. The critical features in this handout are the concepts stressed at the beginning of the session: (1) thinking ahead and developing a strategy of child management, and (2) assigning planned activities for the child to perform during the trip.

There are four elementary parts to this "think aloud–think ahead" method, as follows:

1. *Stop before entering any public place and establish the rules that the child is expected to follow in that place.* At first, the parent is to stop just in front of the entrance to the public place. Then the parent is to establish three or four rules that the child is to follow in the place; these should be rules the child has previously had trouble obeying. The child is to repeat these rules verbatim before proceeding to the next step. For instance, before entering a store with a young child, the parent may say that the rules are, "Stand close, don't touch, and don't beg!" The child is then to repeat these rules to the parent. On subsequent trips to stores, the parent need only prompt the child to repeat the rules by asking, "What are the rules?" If the child fails to recall them properly, the parent restates them and has the child repeat them again. For older children, these rules might be, "Stay next to me, don't touch anything, and do as I say!" Other rules more appropriate to restaurants, churches, or the homes of others would be substituted for these respective situations.

2. *Establish an incentive for compliance.* For children who are already on the poker chip or point systems, these can be used quite readily to reinforce compliance with the rules established in part 1 above. The parent can merely tell the child that he/she will earn a certain number of points or chips for obeying the rules while in the public place. For very young children not on a token system, the parent can take a small cellophane bag of snack treats to the store for use with the child. The chance to earn the treats should be explained to the child before entering the store. A few parents may wish to promise the child a reward that will be purchased at the end of the trip. If this is to be done, it should be used sparingly so as not to establish the expectation in the child that every trip to a public place will result in such purchases. Whichever method of incentive is employed, it is explained to the child before entering the public place.

3. *Establish a disciplinary response for noncompliance.* The parents are now to review with the child what form of punishment they will employ if the child breaks any of the rules set in part 1, or other rules previously explained to be operative in that public place. Wherever possible, this parental response should be the time out procedure used at home or the removal of tokens, depending on the severity of the rule infraction and whether the child is already on a token system at home. Because no chairs are readily available for time out in public places, parents should be prepared to locate quickly a dull corner of the public place where the child would serve the time out period should misbehavior develop. This can be easily accomplished, as most parents know the arrangement of the stores, restaurants, churches, and other public places that they frequently visit. Again, whichever method is to be used, it is to be clearly explained to the child before entering the public place.

4. *Assign an activity or responsibility for the child to perform.* Planning an activity for the child and assigning it to him/her to perform during the public outing can go a long way toward reducing the occurrence of misbehavior. I call this "setting the stage," as it involves the assignment of a planned activity to the child, which may preclude the development of behavior problems. In a store, this could be asking the child to help the parent find certain articles or aisles in the store where the articles are located, or to help with carrying articles throughout the trip. It could also involve checking items off a shopping list when they are found or pushing the shopping cart if one is being used in the store. Whatever the activity, parents can give some thought to its nature on the way to the public place or even just before entering the place. They might even ask the child what he/she could do to help the parent on the trip. In any event, having a planned activity for the child to perform has been shown substantially to reduce disruptive behavior, which can more readily arise when the child is in unstructured situations with nothing to do.

Upon entering the building, the parent is first to scan the area quickly for a potential time out corner before beginning the purpose for which they came to this place. Then, periodically throughout the trip, the parent should attend to and praise the child for adhering to the rules of the setting and for cooperating with the "planned activity" discussed above. For children on token systems, parents can periodically dispense chips or points to the child throughout the time they remain in the public place. It is crucial that parents not wait until the end of the trip before commenting about the child's performance but that they attend to the child's compliance throughout the trip, providing periodic feedback to the child.

If the parent must implement time out, then the child is immediately taken to a quiet, out-of-the-way corner of the building and told to stand in the corner facing the wall until the parent tells the child he/she can leave. At this point, the procedure to be followed is exactly like that used at home except that the minimum sentence needs to be only 30 seconds or so for each year of the child's chronological age. I have found that shorter intervals of time out are just as effective in public places as are longer intervals at home. This is probably due to the fact that the child is missing a great many interesting activities while in time out in public places and that most children experience embarrassment at being given a time out in such places, which further contributes to its aversiveness and hence its effectiveness.

The parents are to remain near the child during time out but should occupy themselves with some other activity so as not to provide attention to the child during this procedure. As at home, the time out episode ends when the child has (1) served a minimum sentence, (2) become quiet for a few moments, and (3) agreed to comply with the rule that was just violated. If the child leaves time out prematurely, the child is returned to the corner and warned that if he/she leaves time out again, he/she will be fined chips or points in the token program. Rarely do children continue "testing" this situation, but should the child leave time out again without permission, the parents fine the child and return him/her to the time out corner thereafter. If this fails to work, terminate the trip if possible and remove the child to the car to serve the time out period, supervised, of course, by the parent.

Because time out has worked successfully at home for the previous few weeks, when it is threatened for use in public places children come to expect that the parent will indeed implement the procedure and hence rarely challenge parental authority in such public places. When the child does violate the explicit rules set forth in part 1, the parent should fine the child using the chip or point system developed at home. If this fails to work, then implement the time out very quickly and without warning, as the child was already warned before entering the public place. I have found that when children are taught that such parental reactions will be swift and decisive, they rarely violate these rules in public places. For parents who prefer not to use time out with the child, alternatives should be discussed. These can be relying on fines in the token system, removing the child from the store, or threatening to remove a privilege the child might have later in the day.

There will be some places in which time out in the building may not be possible, such as in grocery stores where few if any dull corners exist. In such cases, the parents can implement one of these alternatives. First, determine if the child can be taken swiftly outside the building and placed against a wall to serve the time out there. If not, then a second option is to take the child to the car and have him/her sit on the floor of the back seat of the car or on the back seat itself. The parent remains in the front seat or standing outside next to the car. A third alternative is for the parent to record the child's misbehavior in a notebook explicitly carried by the parent for this purpose. Usually, a small, pocket-sized, spiral notepad serves this purpose well. If this option is to be used, it should be explained to the child in front of the public place. Basically, the method involves having the parent record the incident in the notebook and, immediately upon the family's return home, the child is to serve a minimum sentence in time out for each infraction of rules recorded in the notebook. I have discovered that keeping a picture of the child in the notebook that shows the child sitting in the time out chair at home is a useful device for refreshing the child's memory of time out at home. The picture is shown to the child during the explanation of this method before the parent and child enter the public place. A fourth alternative is to place a light hash mark with an ink pen on the back of the child's hand for each rule violation in the store. As with using the notebook, this method requires that the child serve a minimum sentence in time out for each rule violation so recorded, immediately upon the family's return home from that trip.

Reviewing Use of the Procedure in Various Public Places

You can now select several public places in which the child misbehaves and review with the parents how the four steps above would be used before entering those places. The parents should discuss what rules they would establish for those places in which the child commonly misbehaves. In addition, the parents can discuss what forms of incentives and discipline they might wish to use in those places. You can illustrate the use of the method for a store, a restaurant, a church, and the home of someone they are visiting. The method can also be used prior to setting out on long car trips. In addition to following these steps, during a lengthy car trip parents should also take along various play activities to occupy the children so as to preclude misbehavior developing due to sheer boredom during the trip. In case the children should misbehave, points or chips can be deducted during the trip. If the parent wishes to use time out, then they are to park the car in a safe place off of the major roadway and have the child sit on the floor of the back seat or on the back seat itself for the time out interval. Some parents even remove the child from the car to sit on a floor mat placed on the ground beside the car for this time out period. Time out should not be implemented while the parent is trying to drive the vehicle!

Managing Parental Embarrassment

As in previous sessions, you should discuss with the parents their reactions to the use of this method. One reaction that can greatly impede the effective use of this program in public places is the embarrassment parents believe they will suffer should they implement the method while others are watching them. For most parents, a simple explanation will suffice. This explanation should stipulate that few, if any, behavior problems are likely to develop if the parent will follow the steps discussed above before entering the public place. The odds of a problem developing are further reduced by the parents' use of ongoing attention, praise, and rewards for child compliance in the public place. Even where misbehavior develops, it will often be at a much reduced level of disruption because the parent will respond to it swiftly and decisively before it gets out of hand. All of these are likely to reduce any opportunity for the parent to experience embarrassment from this program.

There are always a few parents, however, who are so overwhelmed with the prospect of such embarrassment that they cannot use the methods described above very effectively. For such parents, you may wish to spend a few sessions at this point utilizing a cognitive therapy approach to coping with such parental feelings, such as that taught in rational–emotive therapy. Two books that I have found useful for parents to review in such cases are *Your Erroneous Zones* (Dyer, 1977) and *A New Guide to Rational Living* (Ellis & Harper, 1975). A short review of rational–emotive therapy methods is available in *Rational–Emotive Therapy in Practice* (Bard, 1980), particularly Chapter 5, on parent–child interactions.

In essence, this approach stresses that maladaptive or unpleasant parental emotions in such circumstances are the result of negative and often overly critical self-statements and self-evaluations, which the parent is making during the interaction with the child. Parents are taught to identify these negative and maladaptive statements and to substitute positive coping self-statements in such situations instead. Sometimes, parents may need to record their thoughts in a public place should they experience serious emotional upset over having to deal with their child's behavior. These notes can then be reviewed as part of therapy, and positive coping statements can be designed by the therapist for use by the parent in subsequent encounters with the child's misbehavior in public.

Anticipating Misbehavior across Transitions in Major Activities

This four-step think aloud–think ahead program can be used just as effectively before any situation in which parents anticipate encountering problems with their child. The capacity to generalize these four steps to other activity transitions should be mentioned by the therapist. For instance, at home just before company is about to arrive for dinner or for a social visit with the family would be an excellent time to engage in these four steps with a child. Here are other transition situations where parents can consider using these steps:

- From playtime or watching television to doing homework

- Before a friend of the child arrives to play

- Before a party the child is having at home

- From playtime or watching television to bedtime or bath time

- Before the child goes outside to play

- Before the child goes to the school bus stop or gets on the school bus

The point of this discussion is to get the parents thinking of many times and places where planning ahead and sharing that plan with the child can reduce or even prevent the occurrence of child misbehavior.

Homework

Parents are to continue all of the methods previously taught in this program. For the next week, the parents are to make two bogus trips to stores or other public places with the sole intent of the trip to be to practice the steps discussed above. Parents may wish to record information about these trips for review by the therapist at the next session.

Because the next step of this program will concentrate on how parents can help improve their children's school behavior, it is necessary to determine if behavior in that setting is a problem. Briefly query the parents about the child's school behavior to determine if it is necessary to proceed to Step 8, which deals with such behavior. If school behavior is not a problem, then the therapist may skip to Step 9 of this program. However, I have found Step 8 to provide useful information for parents of defiant children to learn, even if their children are not currently demonstrating behavioral difficulties at school. These children have a high potential for developing some behavioral problems at school in the future, and so reviewing these procedures with the parents can still be useful in preparing them for such difficulties should school behavioral problems arise. If school behavior problems do exist, determine at this point if you need to contact the teacher(s) directly by telephone to discuss these problems or if sending a new set of behavior rating scales to the teacher via the parent is sufficient. I would suggest that the SSQ and the DBDRS-TF be used for this purpose (see Chapter 2 for instructions and Part III for the forms). Parents could have these forms completed by the teacher and bring the forms back to the next session.

Improving School Behavior from Home: The Daily School Behavior Report Card

Goals

1. To review with parents the nature of any behavior problems the child may be demonstrating at school.

2. To instruct parents in the procedures for implementing a daily school behavior report card for their child.

Materials Required

- Parent Handout for Step 8

  Using a Daily School Behavior Report Card

Step Outline

- Review homework
- Discuss with parents any school behavior problems
- Teach parents the procedures to use in establishing a daily school behavior report card

Homework

- Implement a daily school behavior report card
- Continue previously taught methods

As is customary, the session should begin by reviewing the homework from the last session. In this instance, you should query the parents about any shopping trips or other visits to public places where they may have had a chance to try the think aloud–think ahead procedure for reducing the potential for behavior problems in those places. Make any adjustments to the parents' use of these procedures as seem necessary. Also inquire whether the parents had a chance to try these same four steps at home during transitions between major activities. Again, assist the parents with troubleshooting any problems in the implementation of the steps at home and making adjustments to their use of these steps as needed.

Reviewing the Child's School Behavior

Many defiant children, particularly those with ODD and comorbid ADHD, are likely to be having problems with school conduct, either in the classroom or during free times such as recess, lunch period, or in-class periods of free play. Time should be taken here to discuss with the parents any behavior problems their child may be experiencing in the school setting. You will already be aware of some of these difficulties from your initial assessment of this child both through the parent interview as well as the teacher rating scales recommended for use in Chapter 2 (also provided in Part III). And, as discussed in the previous step, you may wish to have parents get a second set of these behavior rating scales completed by the teacher as homework for the previous step so that you can review them now. You may also have decided to call the child's teacher(s) directly in the interim if such detailed information on school behavior in addition to the rating scales is necessary. This information will determine if teaching Step 8 of the program is even necessary. But even if the child is behaving well at school, I nonetheless strongly advise that Step 8 be covered to prepare parents for dealing with such school behavior problems in the future, should they arise.

Implementing a Daily School Behavior Report Card

Although the major responsibility for dealing with a child's school behavior problems rests with the teacher and other school staff, parents can provide some assistance in this regard. One of the most effective means for doing so, apart from setting up an in-class behavior modification program, is the implementation of a home-based reward program that employs a daily school behavior report card as the means for monitoring the child's behavior across the school day. Such report cards are a convenient and cost-effective means of assisting teachers with the management of children's behavior problems at school. The cards provide a rich source of information on the child's conduct at school each day as well as on the child's homework for that evening. The details of how to establish such a report card are set forth in the parent handout accompanying this step.

As the handout indicates, this procedure involves designing a daily school report card that targets behavioral problems this particular child is experiencing at school. You can employ one of the two cards already formatted for this purpose and provided in this handout. The first page of sample cards is one commonly used in my own clinical practice for the past 20 years, targeting the most common areas of behavior in which defiant children are likely to be having difficulties. The second page of sample cards is for dealing with aggressive or defiant children during recess and free time periods at school. A blank report card is also provided as the third page of cards in the handout. This can be used to tailor a daily report card that is quite specific to this child's behavioral difficulties. Whichever card you elect to use, photocopy sufficient copies of the form to provide to the family at the end of this session. Note that two copies of each type of report card are provided on a single page. This was done so that, once photocopied, these pages can be cut in half to provide even more copies of the particular card the parents will be employing.

After deciding which card to use or creating a special card unique to this child, review the use of the card with the family. Be sure that the parents understand that a new card is to be completed by the teachers each day. Parents can either send the new card to school with the child each day or provide the child's first-period teacher with multiple blank copies so that he/she can use a new card each school day. In either case, the intent of the card is to have each of the child's teachers evaluate the child after each school subject or class period. This evaluation is done using the numbers 1 (excellent) to 5 (very poor) and having the teacher place a number beside each behavior to be rated using the column for that class period or subject. Additional comments by the teacher can be written on the back of the card for communicating more details about the child's school day to the parents. The teacher is to initial the bottom of his/her column so as to protect against the child forging the ratings. Even then, a few children have been caught forging their teacher's initials as well as creating false ratings (numbers) to give to their parents. Parents should be told to warn the child that they will be reviewing these cards periodically with the child's teacher and so such forgeries will be detected eventually and then severely penalized.

Besides having each teacher rate the child after each class period, the report card can also be used as a vehicle for communicating the night's homework to the parents. Teachers can have the child write the homework assignments on the back of the card, which should be checked by the teacher for accuracy before the teacher rates the child's behavior and initials the card.

As the handout for parents indicates, this card is to be reviewed each evening by the parents upon the child's return home from school or as soon thereafter as possible. Parents are to make positive comments about the good ratings found on the card (1's and 2's) and use this as a basis for providing encouragement to the child for what he/she seems to be doing well in terms of school conduct. Only then should the parents discuss the child's negative ratings (4's and 5's). They can ask the child to give a brief description of what may have led to the poor rating. More importantly, they can ask what the child might propose to do differently the next school day to improve his/her behavior and ratings. The next school morning, before the child departs for school with a new card, parents should be sure to remind the child of the areas he/she needs to improve.

Following this discussion, points are allocated to each number on the card as noted in the handout: 1 = +25 points (or +5 chips), 2 = +15 points (or +3 chips), 3 = +5 points (or +1 chip), 4 = −15 points (or −3 chips), and 5 = −25 points (or −5 chips). Notice that poor

You should review the attempts of the parents during the previous week(s) in continuing to cope with misbehavior in public places. You should also determine if they have tried using the think aloud–think ahead strategies for major transitions in home activities. Assuming all this has gone well for the family, you can encourage the family to continue to use these same four steps for problems within the home, not just those in public places. There will be many instances where compliance problems with a defiant child are predictable with just a moment's forethought, such as when visitors are in the home, when certain friends of the child come to play, when a party at the home is about to begin, and so forth. Parents can very easily review the four steps taught in prior sessions before these events are about to occur in the home. By doing so, parents will find that such anticipation of and planning for misbehavior greatly increases the likelihood that none will occur. Further examples of how to use these four think aloud–think ahead steps in the home can be provided by you for review with the family, if necessary. Finally, review with the parents their attempts to institute a daily school behavior report card as discussed in the previous session (if that step was presented to the parents). Examine the completed cards brought home from school by the child during the previous 1–2 weeks and discuss how this program seems to be working. Correct any problems with the procedures as needed.

Although this review session and the 1-month booster session are usually the last sessions of the program, some therapists may wish to conduct a few more sessions beyond these to see how well the daily school report card and other management methods are being implemented by the family. Otherwise, a review of these activities can be done at the 1-month booster session that follows Step 9. In other words, this need not be the concluding session of parent training should the therapist believe that greater rehearsal and implementation of the methods of the program are required by a particular family.

Distribute and Review Parent Handout

The parent handout for this session is self-explanatory, and so it will receive little comment here. Basically, it reviews the procedures that parents have been following throughout the course of training and how these might be applied to a new misbehavior, should one develop with the child. The handout explains how parents are to begin keeping a record of the new misbehavior, reviewing that record after 7–10 days to see if it reveals common mistakes to which the parents may have returned, now that parent training is completed. This is followed by the parents' correcting any mistakes they have detected. If this fails to improve the behavior, then the parents are to establish both an incentive and a disciplinary program for this particular behavior problem. Usually, this involves using privileges or a token system as rewards and response cost or time out as the punishment. Stress that using such consequences immediately and consistently is the key to gaining control over any new misbehavior. Parents are to continue keeping a record of the problem behavior throughout this time. If the misbehavior still fails to decline, then they should schedule another appointment with you, being sure to bring along their notes for your review.

Challenging Parents with Hypothetical Behavior Problems

One of the major goals of this session is to begin to wean the parents from dependence on you as the individual who is to solve the child's behavior problems. The parents now have all the skills necessary to cope with the vast majority of behavior problems displayed by most children. Their task now is to begin thinking how they might use these skills in managing any future misbehavior that might arise. You can pose hypothetical behavior problems for the family and request them to think about how they would approach the treatment of these problems using the skills and methods they have acquired in the training program. You can assist where necessary, but this should be done sparingly. Instead, questioning the parents in a Socratic style may help lead them to the correct use of a procedure while fostering their independence from you. Watch for and take care to correct the natural tendency of parents to drift toward punishment methods alone as the first means of dealing with any new behavior problem you pose to them. Continue stressing the principle of "positives before negatives" (rewards before punishments) when designing a behavior change strategy to use with their child.

Homework

There is generally no homework for this session, although you may wish to assign as homework the use of the think aloud–think ahead steps for an in-home child behavior problem. This would be reviewed with the parents in a subsequent session, perhaps the booster session discussed below. If the child has been placed on the daily school behavior report card system, then this should be continued until the booster session 1 month from now, at which time you will review its success.

Booster Session and Follow-Up Meetings

Goals

1. To review parents' implementation of all previously taught procedures and make corrections as needed.

2. To consider whether or not to continue the home token system.

3. To review the use of the daily school behavior report card and make plans for its discontinuation, when appropriate.

4. To discuss any need the child may have for adjunctive psychopharmacological treatment and make appropriate referrals for such treatment.

5. To reassess the nature and degree of the child's disruptive behavior disorders at posttreatment.

Materials Required

- Home Situations Questionnaire
- Disruptive Behavior Disorders Rating Scale—Parent Form

Step Outline

- Review the parents' continuing use of behavior management methods
- Make corrections to management methods as needed
- Consider discontinuation of the token system
- Discuss when and how to phase out the daily school behavior report card
- Consider child's need for adjunctive psychopharmacological treatment and make appropriate referral for it, if needed

At the conclusion of Step 9, you should have scheduled a 1-month booster session if further weekly meetings with the parents were not required. This booster meeting will be used to review some of the general principles taught in the program, to go over any methods about which the parents have questions, and to see how well the family is continuing to implement the procedures of the program. At this point, the parents would complete the posttreatment rating scales (HSQ and DBDRS-PF).

In particular, some discussion may be needed at this point as to how to discontinue the token system. The token system cannot be discontinued completely, however, if the child is on a daily school behavior report card that is linked to home privileges. If the child is not on such a report card, then discontinuation of the token system can take place as need be. As discussed in the session on token systems (Step 4), parents can be told to instruct the child that the token system is being suspended for a few days. However, the child will still earn privileges based on how he/she behaves. Only the record keeping is being discontinued. If the child continues to behave well, the parents will permit the child to have access to daily privileges; if not, some of those privileges will be lost that day depending on the nature of any behavior problems the child may demonstrate. Parents should stress that privileges continue to be linked to appropriate behavior and performance of chores or tasks in the home. Should misbehavior redevelop, the token system can be reinstituted.

For children on a daily school behavior report card, parents should be told to continue using the card daily until the child is able to complete 2 full weeks of school with no ratings of 4 or 5 on the cards. At this point, the use of the card can be reduced to Wednesdays and Fridays. In doing so, the Wednesday card is to be a summary of the child's behavioral performance for Monday through Wednesday, and the Friday card is to cover the child's behavior for Thursday and Friday of that week. If the child goes another 2 full school weeks under this method with no 4's or 5's on the card, then the use of the card is further reduced to a Friday evaluation only. This evaluation would cover the entire school week. Once again, if the child is able to complete another 2 weeks of school on this weekly report card with no ratings of 4 or 5, use of the card can be discontinued. However, the child should be told that if feedback is received from the teachers at school that behavior problems have recurred, then the behavior report card will be used again.

The final point of discussion for some families may be their children's need for adjunctive treatment with psychopharmacology. In particular, children with ADHD will continue to manifest symptoms of this disorder following parent training. If such children have not already been placed on medication for their disorder and the level of their symptoms continues to cause impairment in their home, school, or social functioning, then referral to a physician for consideration of medication treatment may be in order. The most common medications used with ADHD children are the stimulants. However, some antidepressants and antihypertensives may also be of help to certain subgroups of ADHD children. Defiant children who continue to manifest significant mood or anxiety disorders may also require adjunctive medication treatment. This may be the most appropriate time to discuss the need for medication with the parents, if it was not addressed with them before now and assuming such treatments are indicated. Therapists wishing to learn more about medications for ADHD can consult my textbook on that subject (Barkley, 1990), as well as the text by Werry and Aman (1993). Parents wishing more information about such medications may wish to consult my book for parents of ADHD children (Barkley, 1995). The Werry and Aman textbook is also excellent for a review of medications for other childhood disorders.

As this final session concludes, some therapists find it helpful to schedule a second booster session 3–6 months after this, for further monitoring of the family's progress with the procedures. Throughout these follow-up intervals, the family can be encouraged to call you for assistance should it be required.

Congratulations! You have just taken your first family or families through an effective child behavior management training program. Most families will have shown a significant degree of improvement, as reflected both in their verbal comments to you and in declining scores on the HSQ and DBDRS-PF rating scales that you have been readministering periodically across training. If, after using this program, you have suggestions that might help further improve its efficacy, I would welcome them. They can be sent to me by way of the publisher: The Guilford Press, 72 Spring Street, New York, NY 10012.

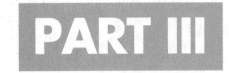
PART III

Assessment Materials

The following instruments are to be used in the evaluation of children referred to mental health professionals where defiant, oppositional, or disruptive behaviors are a major concern involved in the referral of the child. The General Instructions (Form 1) are to be sent to the parent with the Disruptive Behavior Disorders Rating Scale—Parent Form (Form 4), the Home Situations Questionnaire (Form 6), and any other rating scales you wish to have the parent complete about the child, such as the Child Behavior Checklist or Behavioral Assessment System for Children, discussed earlier. Included with this packet of scales should also be the Child and Family Information Form (Form 2) and the Developmental and Medical History Form (Form 3).

Teachers should be mailed a separate packet of rating scales that includes the Disruptive Behavior Disorders Rating Scale—Teacher Form (Form 5), the School Situations Questionnaire (Form 7), and other scales you may want the teacher to complete about the child, such as the Child Behavior Checklist—Teacher Report Form or the Behavioral Assessment System for Children (Teacher Form), as discussed earlier.

Typically, once these scales are returned, a formal appointment with the parents and child will be scheduled, and the parents should be sent the handout on How to Prepare for Your Child's Evaluation (Form 8).

Once the family arrives for the appointment, the clinician should use the Clinical Interview—Parent Report Form (Form 9) in interviewing the parents about the child. This form is filled out by the clinician by asking the parent for the relevant information. Instructions to the interviewer are given in square brackets throughout. Once that interview is completed, the examiner can interview the child while the parents complete rating scales about themselves in the waiting room. These scales might include the Adult Behavior Rating Scales (Forms 10 and 11) as well as any other scales you wish to use, such as the Symptom Checklist 90, the Locke–Wallace Marital Adjustment Scale, the Parenting Stress Index, or others discussed earlier.

Instructions for the use of the above-mentioned instruments are to be found in Part I of this manual.

The General Instructions (Form 1) and the Developmental and Medical History Form (Form 3) were developed by my colleagues in the ADHD Clinic at the University of Massachusetts Medical Center, Arthur Anastopoulos, PhD, George DuPaul, PhD, Terri Shelton, PhD, and Gwenyth Edwards, PhD, as well as by myself. The Clinical Interview (Form 9) found here is updated and adapted from an earlier clinical interview to be found in my text on ADHD (Barkley, 1990). Portions of this interview were also adapted from interviews used previously in our ADHD and Children's Psychopharmacology Clinics at the University of Massachusetts Medical Center. Those interviews were constructed with the assistance of my colleagues, Arthur Anastopoulos, PhD, Daniel Connor, MD, George DuPaul, PhD, Terri Shelton, PhD, and Gwenyth Edwards, PhD. I am most grateful for their permitting me to adapt portions of those interviews to include in the present one. The other rating scales and the brochure for preparing children for an evaluation to be found here were developed by me explicitly for this manual.

The author and publisher grant permission for the purchaser of this manual to photocopy these assessment materials solely for use in the purchaser's professional practice and solely for the evaluation of children under the professional care of the purchaser (see the copyright page for details).

The forms included in this section also appear in a Spanish-language supplement available from the publisher.

Contents of Part III

General Instructions for Completing the Questionnaires (Form 1) — 169

Child and Family Information Form (Form 2) — 170

Developmental and Medical History Form (Form 3) — 171

Disruptive Behavior Disorders Rating Scale—Parent Form (Form 4) — 174

Disruptive Behavior Disorders Rating Scale—Teacher Form (Form 5) — 176

Home Situations Questionnaire (Form 6) — 177

School Situations Questionnaire (Form 7) — 178

How to Prepare for Your Child's Evaluation (Form 8) — 179

Clinical Interview—Parent Report Form (Form 9) — 188

Adult Behavior Rating Scale—Self-Report of Current Behavior (Form 10) — 213

Adult Behavior Rating Scale—Self-Report of Childhood Behavior (Form 11) — 214

GENERAL INSTRUCTIONS
FOR COMPLETING THE QUESTIONNAIRES (FORM 1)

As part of processing your request for an evaluation of your child at our clinic, we must ask you to complete the enclosed forms about your child and your family. We greatly appreciate your willingness to complete these forms. Your answers will give us a much better understanding of your child's behavior at home and your family circumstances. In completing these forms, please follow these instructions as closely as possible:

1. *All* forms in this packet should be completed by the parent who has the primary responsibility for caring for this child. Where both parents reside with the child, this is to be the parent who spends the greatest amount of time with the child.

2. If a second parent wishes to complete a second packet of information about this child, he/she may do so independently by requesting a second set of these forms. He/she may call our administrative assistant, _____, at _____ (phone), and the packet will be sent out promptly.

3. If your child is already taking medication for assistance with his/her behavior management (such as Ritalin) or for any emotional difficulties (such as an antidepressant), we must ask that you complete the questionnaires about your child's behavior *based on how your child behaves when he/she is OFF this medication*. It is very likely that you occasionally observe your child's behavior at periods when he/she is off of this medication, and we want you to use those time periods to answer these questions about behavior. In this way, we can get a clearer idea of the true nature of your child's difficulties without the alterations produced by any medication treatments being used. However, some parents whose children have been on medication for a long time may not be able to give us this information. In that case, just complete the questionnaires based on your child's behavior, but check the third blank line below to let us know that you based your judgments on your child's behavior when he/she was on medication. Check one of the blanks below to let us know for certain on what basis you judged your child's behavior in answering our behavior questionnaires:

   —— My child currently does *not* take any medication for behavior problems. My answers are based on my child's behavior while he/she is off of medication.
   —— My child *is currently taking medication* for behavior problems. However, my answers are based on my child's behavior while he/she is *OFF* of this medication.
   —— My child *is currently taking medication* for behavior problems. My answers are based on my child's behavior while he/she is *ON* this medication.

If your child is currently taking medication for behavioral or emotional difficulties, please list these medications below:

_____

Thank you for completing these forms and returning them promptly to us in the enclosed envelope.

PLEASE RETURN THIS FORM ALONG WITH THE COMPLETED QUESTIONNAIRES.

CHILD AND FAMILY INFORMATION (FORM 2)

Child's name _____ **Birthdate** _____ **Age** _____

Address _____
                (Street)   (City)   (State)   (Zip)

Home phone ( ) _____ Work phone ( ) _____ Dad/Mom
                                                                    (Circle one)

Child's school _____ Teacher's name _____

School address _____
                (Street)   (City)   (State)   (Zip)

School phone ( ) _____ Child's grade _____

Is child in special education? Yes No If so, what type? _____

Father's name _____ Age _____ Education _____
                                                                     (Years)

Father's place of employment _____

Type of employment _____ Annual salary _____

Mother's name _____ Age _____ Education _____
                                                                      (Years)

Mother's place of employment _____

Type of employment _____ Annual salary _____

Is child adopted? Yes No If yes, age when adopted _____

Are parents married? Yes No Separated? Yes No Divorced? Yes No

Child's physician _____

Physician's address _____
                  (Street)   (City)   (State)   (Zip)

Physician's telephone number _____

Please list all other children in the family:

Name	Age	School grade

DEVELOPMENTAL AND MEDICAL HISTORY (FORM 3)

PREGNANCY AND DELIVERY

A. Length of pregnancy (e.g., full term, 40 weeks, 32 weeks, etc.) _____

B. Length of delivery (number of hours from initial labor pains to birth) _____

C. Mother's age when child was born _____

D. Child's birth weight _____

E. Did any of the following conditions occur during pregnancy/delivery?

1. Bleeding	No	Yes
2. Excessive weight gain (more than 30 lbs.)	No	Yes
3. Toxemia/preeclampsia	No	Yes
4. Rh factor incompatibility	No	Yes
5. Frequent nausea or vomiting	No	Yes
6. Serious illness or injury	No	Yes
7. Took prescription medications a. If yes, name of medication _____	No	Yes
8. Took illegal drugs	No	Yes
9. Used alcoholic beverage a. If yes, approximate number of drinks per week ____	No	Yes

10. Smoked cigarettes
    a. If yes, approximate number of cigarettes per day
    (e.g., ½ pack) _____
	No	Yes

11. Was given medication to ease labor pains a. If yes, name of medication _____	No	Yes
12. Delivery was induced	No	Yes
13. Forceps were used during delivery	No	Yes
14. Had a breech delivery	No	Yes
15. Had a cesarean section delivery	No	Yes
16. Other problems—please describe	No	Yes

F. Did any of the following conditions affect your child during delivery or within the first few days after birth?

1. Injured during delivery	No	Yes
2. Cardiopulmonary distress during delivery	No	Yes

(cont.)

3. Delivered with cord around neck	No	Yes
4. Had trouble breathing following delivery	No	Yes
5. Needed oxygen	No	Yes
6. Was cyanotic, turned blue	No	Yes
7. Was jaundiced, turned yellow	No	Yes
8. Had an infection	No	Yes
9. Had seizures	No	Yes
10. Was given medications	No	Yes
11. Born with a congenital defect	No	Yes
12. Was in hospital more than 7 days	No	Yes

INFANT HEALTH AND TEMPERAMENT

A. During the first 12 months, was your child:

1. Difficult to feed	No	Yes
2. Difficult to get to sleep	No	Yes
3. Colicky	No	Yes
4. Difficult to put on a schedule	No	Yes
5. Alert	No	Yes
6. Cheerful	No	Yes
7. Affectionate	No	Yes
8. Sociable	No	Yes
9. Easy to comfort	No	Yes
10. Difficult to keep busy	No	Yes
11. Overactive, in constant motion	No	Yes
12. Very stubborn, challenging	No	Yes

EARLY DEVELOPMENTAL MILESTONES

A. At what age did your child first accomplish the following:
1. Sitting without help _____
2. Crawling _____
3. Walking alone, without assistance _____
4. Using single words (e.g.,"mama," "dada," "ball", etc.) _____
5. Putting two or more words together (e.g.,"mama up") _____

(cont.)

6. Bowel training, day and night   _____
7. Bladder training, day and night   _____

HEALTH HISTORY

A. Date of child's last physical exam: _____

B. At any time has your child had the following:

1. Asthma	Never	Past	Present
2. Allergies	Never	Past	Present
3. Diabetes, arthritis, or other chronic illnesses	Never	Past	Present
4. Epilepsy or seizure disorder	Never	Past	Present
5. Febrile seizures	Never	Past	Present
6. Chicken pox or other common childhood illnesses	Never	Past	Present
7. Heart or blood pressure problems	Never	Past	Present
8. High fevers (over 103°)	Never	Past	Present
9. Broken bones	Never	Past	Present
10. Severe cuts requiring stitches	Never	Past	Present
11. Head injury with loss of consciousness	Never	Past	Present
12. Lead poisoning	Never	Past	Present
13. Surgery	Never	Past	Present
14. Lengthy hospitalization	Never	Past	Present
15. Speech or language problems	Never	Past	Present
16. Chronic ear infections	Never	Past	Present
17. Hearing difficulties	Never	Past	Present
18. Eye or vision problems	Never	Past	Present
19. Fine motor/handwriting problems	Never	Past	Present
20. Gross motor difficulties, clumsiness	Never	Past	Present
21. Appetite problems (overeating or undereating)	Never	Past	Present
22. Sleep problems (falling asleep, staying asleep)	Never	Past	Present
23. Soiling problems	Never	Past	Present
24. Wetting problems	Never	Past	Present

25. Other health difficulties—please describe

DISRUPTIVE BEHAVIOR DISORDERS RATING SCALE—PARENT FORM (FORM 4)

Child's name_____ Age_____ Date_____

Form completed by: _____

Relationship to child: (Circle one)

    Mother   Father   Stepparent   Other:_____ (explain)

Instructions: Circle the number that *best describes* your child's behavior at home over the past 6 months.

	Never or rarely	Sometimes	Often	Very often
1. Fails to give close attention to details or makes careless mistakes in schoolwork	0	1	2	3
2. Has difficulty sustaining attention in tasks or play activities	0	1	2	3
3. Does not seem to listen when spoken to directly	0	1	2	3
4. Does not follow through on instructions and fails to finish work	0	1	2	3
5. Has difficulty organizing tasks and activities	0	1	2	3
6. Avoids tasks (e.g., schoolwork, homework) that require mental effort	0	1	2	3
7. Loses things necessary for tasks or activities	0	1	2	3
8. Is easily distracted	0	1	2	3
9. Is forgetful in daily activities	0	1	2	3
10. Fidgets with hands or feet or squirms in seat	0	1	2	3
11. Leaves seat in classroom or in other situations in which remaining seated is expected	0	1	2	3
12. Runs about or climbs excessively in situations in which it is inappropriate	0	1	2	3
13. Has difficulty playing or engaging in leisure activities quietly	0	1	2	3
14. Is "on the go" or acts as if "driven by a motor"	0	1	2	3
15. Talks excessively	0	1	2	3
16. Blurts out answers before questions have been completed	0	1	2	3
17. Has difficulty awaiting turn	0	1	2	3

(cont.)

	Never or rarely	Sometimes	Often	Very often
18. Interrupts or intrudes on others	0	1	2	3
19. Loses temper	0	1	2	3
20. Argues with adults	0	1	2	3
21. Actively defies or refuses to comply with adults' requests or rules	0	1	2	3
22. Deliberately annoys people	0	1	2	3
23. Blames others for his/her mistakes or misbehavior	0	1	2	3
24. Is touchy or easily annoyed by others	0	1	2	3
25. Is angry and resentful	0	1	2	3
26. Is spiteful or vindictive	0	1	2	3

Instructions: Please indicate whether your child has done any of these activities in the past 12 months.

1. Often bullied, threatened, or intimidated others	No	Yes
2. Often initiated physical fights	No	Yes
3. Used a weapon that can cause serious physical harm to others (e.g., a bat, brick, broken bottle, knife, or gun)	No	Yes
4. Has been physically cruel to people	No	Yes
5. Has been physically cruel to animals	No	Yes
6. Has stolen while confronting a victim (e.g., mugging, purse snatching, extortion, armed robbery)	No	Yes
7. Has forced someone into sexual activity	No	Yes
8. Has deliberately engaged in fire setting with the intention of causing serious damage	No	Yes
9. Has deliberately destroyed others' property (other than by fire setting)	No	Yes
10. Has broken into someone else's house, building, or car	No	Yes
11. Often lies to obtain goods or favors or to avoid obligations (i.e., "cons" others)	No	Yes
12. Has stolen items of nontrivial value without confronting a victim (e.g., shoplifting, but without breaking and entering; forgery)	No	Yes
13. Often stays out at night despite parental prohibitions If so, at what age did this begin?____	No	Yes
14. Has run away from home overnight at least twice while living in parent's home, foster care, or group home. If so, how many times?____	No	Yes
15. Is often truant from school If so, at what age did he/she begin doing this?____	No	Yes

DISRUPTIVE BEHAVIOR DISORDERS RATING SCALE—TEACHER FORM (FORM 5)

Child's name_____ **Date** _____

Form completed by _____

Approximately how many hours are you with this child each school day?_____

What subject(s) do you regularly teach this child? _____

Instructions: Circle the number that *best describes* this child's behavior at school during the past 6 months.

	Never or rarely	Sometimes	Often	Very often
1. Fails to give close attention to details or makes careless mistakes in schoolwork	0	1	2	3
2. Has difficulty sustaining attention in tasks or play activities	0	1	2	3
3. Does not seem to listen when spoken to directly	0	1	2	3
4. Does not follow through on instructions and fails to finish work	0	1	2	3
5. Has difficulty organizing tasks and activities	0	1	2	3
6. Avoids tasks (e.g., schoolwork, homework) that require mental effort	0	1	2	3
7. Loses things necessary for tasks or activities	0	1	2	3
8. Is easily distracted	0	1	2	3
9. Is forgetful in daily activities	0	1	2	3
10. Fidgets with hands or feet or squirms in seat	0	1	2	3
11. Leaves seat in classroom or in other situations in which remaining seated is expected	0	1	2	3
12. Runs about or climbs excessively in situations in which it is inappropriate	0	1	2	3
13. Has difficulty playing or engaging in leisure activities quietly	0	1	2	3
14. Is "on the go" or acts as if "driven by a motor"	0	1	2	3
15. Talks excessively	0	1	2	3
16. Blurts out answers before questions have been completed	0	1	2	
17. Has difficulty awaiting turn	0	1	2	3
18. Interrupts or intrudes on others	0	1	2	3
19. Loses temper	0	1	2	3
20. Argues with adults	0	1	2	3
21. Actively defies or refuses to comply with adults' requests or rules	0	1	2	3
22. Deliberately annoys people	0	1	2	3
23. Blames others for his/her mistakes or misbehavior	0	1	2	3
24. Is touchy or easily annoyed by others	0	1	2	3
25. Is angry and resentful	0	1	2	3
26. Is spiteful or vindictive	0	1	2	3

HOME SITUATIONS QUESTIONNAIRE (FORM 6)

Child's name_____ Date_____

Name of person completing this form_____

Instructions: Does your child present any problems with compliance to instructions, commands, or rules for you in any of these situations? If so, please circle the word Yes and then circle a number beside that situation that describes how severe the problem is for you. If your child is not a problem in a situation, circle No and go on to the next situation on the form.

Situations	Yes/No		Mild			If yes, how severe?				Severe	
While playing alone	Yes	No	1	2	3	4	5	6	7	8	9
While playing with other children	Yes	No	1	2	3	4	5	6	7	8	9
At mealtimes	Yes	No	1	2	3	4	5	6	7	8	9
Getting dressed	Yes	No	1	2	3	4	5	6	7	8	9
Washing and bathing	Yes	No	1	2	3	4	5	6	7	8	9
While you are on the telephone	Yes	No	1	2	3	4	5	6	7	8	9
While watching television	Yes	No	1	2	3	4	5	6	7	8	9
When visitors are in your home	Yes	No	1	2	3	4	5	6	7	8	9
When you are visiting someone's home	Yes	No	1	2	3	4	5	6	7	8	9
In public places (restaurants, stores, church, etc.)	Yes	No	1	2	3	4	5	6	7	8	9
When father is home	Yes	No	1	2	3	4	5	6	7	8	9
When asked to do chores	Yes	No	1	2	3	4	5	6	7	8	9
When asked to do homework	Yes	No	1	2	3	4	5	6	7	8	9
At bedtime	Yes	No	1	2	3	4	5	6	7	8	9
While in the car	Yes	No	1	2	3	4	5	6	7	8	9
When with a babysitter	Yes	No	1	2	3	4	5	6	7	8	9

- For Office Use Only -

Total number of problem settings_____ Mean severity score_____

SCHOOL SITUATIONS QUESTIONNAIRE (FORM 7)

Child's name_____ Date_____

Name of person completing this form_____

Instructions: Does this child present any problems with compliance to instructions, commands, or rules for you in any of these situations? If so, please circle the word Yes and then circle a number beside that situation that describes how severe the problem is for you. If this child is not a problem in a situation, circle No and go on to the next situation on the form.

Situations	Yes/No		Mild				If yes, how severe?				Severe
When arriving at school	Yes	No	1	2	3	4	5	6	7	8	9
During individual desk work	Yes	No	1	2	3	4	5	6	7	8	9
During small group activities	Yes	No	1	2	3	4	5	6	7	8	9
During free playtime in class	Yes	No	1	2	3	4	5	6	7	8	9
During lectures to the class	Yes	No	1	2	3	4	5	6	7	8	9
At recess	Yes	No	1	2	3	4	5	6	7	8	9
At lunch	Yes	No	1	2	3	4	5	6	7	8	9
In the hallways	Yes	No	1	2	3	4	5	6	7	8	9
In the bathroom	Yes	No	1	2	3	4	5	6	7	8	9
On field trips	Yes	No	1	2	3	4	5	6	7	8	9
During special assemblies	Yes	No	1	2	3	4	5	6	7	8	9
On the bus	Yes	No	1	2	3	4	5	6	7	8	9

- For Office Use Only -

Total number of problem settings_____ Mean severity score_____

HOW TO PREPARE FOR YOUR CHILD'S EVALUATION (FORM 8)

Taking your child to a mental health professional for an evaluation is a major decision for any parent. Many parents do not know what to expect from such an evaluation and what they can do to be well prepared for it. That is why we are sending this pamphlet to you. It will give you some idea of how to prepare for your child's evaluation so that the time you spend with the professional can be used to its maximum advantage.

GETTING READY

In deciding to seek our professional help, consider what your concerns are at the moment. Typically, these concerns reflect problems with your child's behavioral, emotional, family, school, or social adjustment. While waiting for the appointment date, take time to sit down with a sheet of paper and make up a list of answers to the following questions in areas that may be of concern to you. This can help clarify your thoughts about your child's difficulties. It can also make the evaluation proceed more smoothly and quickly, perhaps even saving time (and money) in the process (professionals usually charge by the quarter hour for their time). Here are the areas to consider:

1. What most concerns you now about your child? Don't go into a long explanation, just list the major problem areas. It helps to identify first of all whether they are mainly problems at home, in school, in the neighborhood or community, or with other children, or in all of these areas. Use these areas as headings on your list. To help a professional help you, it is important that you get down to specifics. What precisely is it that you are concerned about with your child in these areas? Underneath "Home Problems," jot down those problem behaviors that you think are inappropriate for your child's age. That is, these problems seem to occur more often or to a degree that is beyond what you think to be typical of normal children at this age. Even if you do not think they are deviant for your child's age, if you are concerned about them anyway, write them down but indicate this fact next to that item. Now do the same for "School Problems" and the rest of these problem headings (Neighborhood, Peers, and other problem areas). Save this list to take with you to your appointment with the professional.

2. Now on the back of that sheet of paper, or on a new sheet if that one is full, write down these major headings and list anything that comes to mind that your child has difficulties with that might indicate a problem in these areas: Health (chronic or recurring medical problems), Intelligence or Mental Development, Motor Development and Coordination, Problems with Senses (such as eyesight, hearing, etc.), Academic Learning Abilities (such as reading, math, etc.), Anxiety or Fears, Depression, Aggression toward Others, Hyperactivity, Poor Attention, and Antisocial Behavior (such as lying, stealing, setting fires, running away from home, etc.). You may already have listed some of these in #1 above, but it can help to reorganize them into these new categories for your child's professional evaluation.

(cont.)

3. Some parents may have concerns that they are embarrassed to raise with professionals. These often involve family problems that the parents believe may be contributing to their child's behavioral or emotional problems, but which they are reluctant to divulge to others. Such problems as alcoholism or substance abuse in one of the parents, marital problems that create frequent conflicts between the parents and may spill over into mistreatment of the child, episodes of excessive disciplining or physical punishment that may indicate abuse of the child, and suspected sexual abuse of the child are just some of the many areas parents may be hesitant to divulge to a professional who is a stranger to them. But parents should realize that these are extremely important matters for the mental health professional to understand and take into consideration in attempting to diagnose and treat children. If this information is withheld, then there will be an increased possibility of mistakes in diagnosis, the formulation of the important issues in the case, and treatment planning, because the professional is being intentionally kept in the dark about matters that have a direct bearing on a complete understanding of the case.

4. If at all possible, speak with your child's teacher(s) and write down what they tell you they are most concerned about with your child's school adjustment. Again, save this list to take with you to your child's professional appointment.

5. Now take one more sheet of paper and make a list of any problems you think are occurring in your family besides those of your child. Use the following headings if it will help: *Personal* problems (things you think are troubling you about yourself), *marital* problems, problems with *money*, problems with *relatives*, problems related to your *job* or that of your spouse, problems with *other children* in the family, and *health* problems that you or your spouse may have. Take this list with you to your appointment.

These lists are similar to the areas most likely to be covered in the interview the professional has with you. Keep the lists handy around your home and add items to them as you think of them while waiting for the professional appointment. These lists should help to focus the evaluation quickly on the most important areas of concern that you have about your child and your family. They will also probably help speed up the evaluation and keep things on track. Making these lists probably will help you clarify your own thinking about your current situation and your child's problems. Finally, these lists will help to maximize the usefulness of the evaluation for you and your child. This may result in the professional having greater respect and appreciation for you, a consumer who has come in well prepared for the evaluation.

THE EVALUATION

The clinical interview with you, the parents (and to a lesser extent, with your child), is probably the most important component of a comprehensive professional evaluation of a child. Other important elements are your completed behavior questionnaires about your child, an interview with your child's teacher(s), and similar behavior questionnaires about the child completed by his/her teacher(s).

(cont.)

What Information Will We Need from You to Do the Evaluation?

Plenty! Before professionals can identify or diagnose a child as having behavioral, emotional, or learning problems, they must collect a great deal of information about the child and family, sift through this information looking for the presence of any psychological disorders, determine how serious the problems are likely to be, rule out or rule in other disorders or problems the child might have, and consider what resources are available in your area to deal with these problems. If your child also needs educational or psychological testing for any learning or developmental problems he/she may be having besides the behavior problems, this will be discussed with you on the day of your appointment, and you will be referred to another psychologist or educational specialist for this additional evaluation. You can expect our evaluation to run an average of 2.5–4 hours.

What Else Is Needed to Complete the Evaluation?

Many times our professionals need information from others who know your child, in addition to the information you will give us. You may be asked to (1) give your permission for the professional to get the reports of previous evaluations that your child may have been given; (2) permit the professional to contact your child's treating physician for further information on health status and medication treatment, if any; (3) provide the results of the most recent educational evaluation from your child's school; (4) initiate one of these school evaluations, if one was not already done and if one of your concerns is your child's school adjustment; (5) complete the packet of behavior questionnaires about your child that should have been sent to you earlier by mail; (6) return these forms before the appointment date; (7) give your permission to have your child's teacher(s) complete similar behavior questionnaires, which will be mailed to them; and (8) give permission for the professional to obtain any information from social service agencies that already may be involved in providing services to your child.

There is rarely any reason for you to deny our professionals your permission to obtain the above information from others or for you to refuse to institute the procedures requested of you. However, on rare occasions, you may wish an unbiased second opinion about your child's problems. This may happen if you have already had an evaluation by the school or another professional with which you strongly disagree. In such cases, you may wish to tell us not to obtain the records from the other professional or from any school evaluation. Should you do so, please explain why you are withholding your permission for the release of these particular sources of information so that we have a clearer grasp of the issues involved in your request for this new evaluation with us. However, in most cases you should not deny our professionals access to the information that can be provided by your child's teachers, even if you disagree with those teachers. Preventing professionals from speaking with your child's teachers greatly diminishes the ability of those professionals to understand your child. It precludes their getting information from the second most important caregiver in your child's current situation. If you disagree with what a teacher may say, explain this to the professionals before they contact the school so they can keep this disagreement in mind as they speak with the teacher.

(cont.)

What Happens on the Day of the Appointment?

Several things. You are going to be interviewed for about 1–2 hours about your child, and your child most likely will be interviewed as well. It is the interview with you that is most important. You probably are going to be asked to complete some behavior questionnaires as well, if you were not sent any to complete before the appointment. Your child may also be tested if there are issues to be answered about his/her intelligence, language and academic skills, or other mental abilities (such as memory, motor skills, etc.).

The Parent Interview

The interview with you, the parent, is an indispensable part of the evaluation of your child. No adult is more likely to have the wealth of knowledge about, the history of interactions with, or simply the time spent with a child than you. Whenever possible, both parents should attend the interview, as they each have a somewhat unique perspective on the child's problems. If employment or other reasons preclude one parent from attending, the other parent should speak with the partner the day before the evaluation and write down that parent's concerns and opinions about the child to take into the evaluation the next day. It is usually not necessary that brothers and sisters attend this first evaluation. In some cases, the professional may request that these siblings attend a second meeting if the professional feels it is necessary to get the siblings' view of particular family conflicts or problems the siblings are having with the child being evaluated.

The interview with you serves several purposes. First, it establishes an important relationship between you and the professional and even between the child and the professional, which will be helpful and put you at ease with the rest of the evaluation. Second, the interview provides an important source of invaluable information about your child and family. In particular, it gives the professional your view of your child's apparent problems and narrows the focus of later stages of the evaluation. This is your chance to get your concerns about your child out in the open with a knowledgeable professional. Don't be shy, coy, or unforthcoming. The more information you can provide the professional, the better appreciation he/she can have of your child's problems and the more accurate the diagnosis is likely to be. Use the lists that you constructed while waiting for the appointment date so you don't forget anything you wanted to discuss. Third, the interview can often reveal just how much distress the child's problems are causing you and your family. It also gives the professional some sense of your own well-being as a parent. Fourth, the interview may begin to reveal significant information about your relationship with your child that could be important in pinpointing some potential contributors to your child's problem. But two of the most important purposes of this evaluation are to determine a diagnosis of your child's problem(s) and to provide you with reasonable treatment recommendations.

The professional is likely to make notes throughout the conversation with you. He/she will also jot down his/her own observations of you and how your child is doing while you both are in the clinic. Although these notes from observing you and your child may be helpful in raising certain ideas about your child's problems that can be discussed with you later, they will not be overly emphasized by our professionals. Behavior in the office, particular that of your child, is often not

(cont.)

very helpful in telling us how your child is likely to behave at home or in school. In general, research with children having behavior problems has shown that many are likely to behave normally during this evaluation. Such normal behavior will not be interpreted by our professionals as indicating that your child has no problems. However, if your child displays a lot of inattentive, hyperactive, or defiant behavior during the evaluation, this may be more informative, as such behavior is unusual for normal children and could indicate your child would have similar problems in school.

Some of our professionals like to have your child present during the interview with you. In part, this is to give them some idea of how you and your child get along with each other. This is fine so long as your child is not likely to be upset by the nature of the questions and with your answers about your child. Some parents do not feel comfortable with this situation as they do not want to talk about the child's problems in front of him/her, at least not yet. If you feel that having your child present during the interview would make you inhibited and less candid about your opinions and concerns, then simply advise the professionals politely of your feelings on the matter when you first meet with them the day of the evaluation. It should not be a problem for us to handle things your way.

INFORMATION ABOUT YOUR CHILD

The interview will probably begin with an explanation of the procedures to be undertaken as part of this evaluation and the time it is expected to take. If it has not been discussed already, the estimated cost of the evaluation and the manner in which the fee is to be handled (e.g., insurance, self-pay, etc.) should be discussed with you. Our professionals may point out to you at this time that although most of what you say is confidential (they cannot tell anyone else about what you have said without your permission), laws may place limits on this privilege. These limits are about reports of child neglect or abuse. Where you mention such information to the professional, he/she may be required by law to report this information to the state, usually the Department of Social Services. The clinician will tell you about such limits on the day of your evaluation.

The interview will probably proceed to a discussion of your concerns about your child. You can refer to the notes that you made before the appointment here. You will probably be asked to give some specific examples of your child's behavior that illustrate why you are concerned about it. For instance, if you say that you are worried that your child is too impulsive, you may be asked to give some examples of your child's impulsive behavior. This is done not to challenge your opinion but to help the interviewer see how you arrived at that opinion. Give as much information as you can when asked. You may also be asked how you are presently trying to manage your child's behavior problems and whether your spouse is using a different approach. It is common for behavior problem children to be somewhat better behaved for their fathers than mothers. It is all right to describe such differences as they do not mean you or your spouse are doing anything wrong or are causing the problems with your child.

You are going to be questioned about when you first noticed your child's problems and how long each of the major problem areas has been occurring. Try to be as specific as your memory will permit. Again, taking some notes about this before the appointment may help you to remember

(cont.)

this information better when you are asked. This naturally leads to questions about the types of previous professional assistance you may have obtained and whether it is possible for the interviewer to contact these other professionals for further details about your child and your family. Our professionals like to ask parents what they believe has led their child to develop these problems. If you have an opinion on what caused your child's problems, it is all right to say it, but don't be afraid simply to say you don't know. The professional is just looking to see if you can provide him/her with any additional insight about the cause of your child's difficulties. Remember, we as professionals do not know the exact causes of all children's behavior problems, although we have much information that can be of help to us in narrowing down these possibilities. Sometimes it simply is not possible to say for sure why certain children behave the way they do. Don't feel as though you have to come up with a better explanation for your child's behavior.

If you completed behavior rating forms before the appointment and returned them, the professional may want to review some of your answers with you now, especially those that may have been unclear to him/her. If the professional does not go over your answers with you, *you* may want to ask *the professional* if he/she has any questions about your answers on those forms. You may also be asked about some answers on the forms that were sent to your child's teacher(s). If you are curious, you may ask to see the teacher's answers on these forms. It is your right to see what the teacher has said. Ask the professional to explain anything about these forms and their answers that is confusing to you.

The professional will also talk with you about any problems your child has within a number of different developmental domains. We customarily ask parents about their children's development so far in their physical health, sensory and motor abilities, language, thinking, intellect, academic achievement, self-help skills such as dressing and bathing, social behavior, emotional problems, and family relationships. You will probably be asked about similar things. Many professionals will also review with you a variety of behavior problems or symptoms of other psychiatric problems to see if your child also may be having these difficulties. Simply be truthful and indicate whether or not these other symptoms are present and to what degree.

Because our professionals are trying to evaluate your child's problems, they are likely to spend most or all of the time with you trying to identify the areas of concern you have about your child. This is fine. But our professionals also want to ask you about any strengths your child has in any of the areas discussed above or in particular hobbies, sports, or school subjects. If the professional does not ask you, then mention some yourself to give a more complete and balanced picture of your child to the professional. We also like to take an opportunity to ask parents about possible special interests, privileges, and rewards that your child enjoys. We can typically use this information later if we have to set up a reward program for your child as part of our behavior management training with parents.

At some point in the interview, the professional may review your child's developmental and medical history with you. You will have completed a form about this for us before the appointment, but we may want to review your answers with you as part of the interview.

(*cont.*)

It is essential that the professional discuss with you your child's school history. Many children referred to us have difficulties adjusting to the demands of school. You are likely to be asked about the age at which your child began kindergarten, what school he/she attended, and how well your child progressed through this and subsequent grades and schools. You probably will be questioned about the types of special educational evaluations and placements your child has received, if any, and whether your child had a team evaluation conducted by the school. If one has not been done, you may be asked to initiate one in case your child has school problems that make the child eligible for any formal special educational services. You are also going to be asked about what specific concerns your child's teacher(s) have raised about school performance, both now and in the past. Be sure to tell the professional if your child has repeated a grade, or has been suspended or expelled. We also like to question parents about the nature of the relationship they presently have with the school staff working with their child. Is it friendly and supportive, or filled with conflict? Has communication been open and reasonably clear, or limited and hostile? This greatly helps us in preparing for later contacts with the school staff if these are needed. If the professional forgets to ask about this, you may want to raise the topic yourself to give the professional a clearer picture of your past relations with the school staff.

You may be asked to give written permission for the professional to contact your child's school, if it was not obtained previously from you. You should consent to this under most circumstances, as it is very hard for a professional to evaluate your child's problems fully without access to the school's information. If you do not want this done, be sure to give the professionals a clear explanation as to why you do not, so they do not misjudge you as being unreasonably hostile to them or to the school.

INFORMATION ABOUT YOU AND YOUR FAMILY

Professionals know that many families of behavior problem children are under more stress than other families and that the parents may be having more personal problems than most parents whose children do not have behavior problems. Do not be offended if you are asked such personal questions. Information about you and your family can be of great assistance to the professional in helping to understand your child's problems better and develop more useful treatment recommendations for you. It may also indicate to the interviewer that you may need some additional help for your own or your family's other problems. You will probably be asked about your own background, education, and occupation, as well as those of your spouse. The professional may ask if you or your spouse have had any psychiatric, learning, developmental, or chronic medical problems. Parents are also typically asked during such evaluations whether they are having marital problems and what the nature of these might be. All of these personal questions are routine and important, so please answer as honestly as you can.

We will ask you about other children in the immediate family and any psychological, educational, developmental, or other problems these siblings may be having.

Before the interview with you is over, take a minute to review the notes that you brought with you to see if all of your concerns have been covered with the professional you are seeing. Share with

(cont.)

the professional any further information on these notes or anything else you feel might be helpful in better understanding your child and your family. Your candor and openness will be respected and appreciated by our professional staff.

The Child Interview

Depending on your child's age and intelligence, some time during the evaluation will be spent by the professional in interviewing your child and making some informal observations of your child's appearance, behavior, and developmental skills. This interview serves much the same purposes as the interview with you. However, you should not place too much emphasis on the information we obtain in this interview. Such informal observations of your child's conduct during the interview may not be typical of your child's behavior at home or school, as mentioned earlier. Our professionals will not make the mistake of placing too much weight on the observations of your child in our clinic. Do not be surprised to find that your child is well behaved during this evaluation, and do not worry about it.

Your child is probably going to be asked a lot of general questions. These will probably deal with the following areas:

1. What is your child's awareness of why he/she is visiting the interviewer today and what have the parents told him/her about the reason for the visit?
2. What are the child's favorite hobbies, television shows, sports, or pets?
3. Where does the child attend school, who are his/her teachers, what types of subjects does he/she take in school, and which does he/she like most? If the child is doing poorly in a subject, what reasons does he/she give to explain any such difficulties?
4. Does the child see him/herself as having any behavior problems in the classroom? What types of discipline does the child get from the teacher(s) for any such misconduct?
5. How does the child think he/she is accepted by other children at school?
6. What are your child's perceptions of any of the problems that you have reported to the professional?
7. What would your child like to see changed or improved at home or at school?
8. The professional may then ask your child about whether he/she sees him/herself as having any behavioral problems. If the child does, he/she will likely be asked why and what he/she thinks causes this pattern of behavior.

Our professionals are aware that children are notorious for underreporting their difficulties and are likely to do so in this part of the interview. Thus, the professional will not use your child's answers in determining if the child actually has a behavioral, learning, or emotional disorder.

Some of our professionals find it helpful during this interview, particularly if it is with young children, to let them play, draw, or simply wander about the office. Others may ask them a series of incomplete sentences, letting the children fill in the blanks with their own answers. This can be a less direct way of finding out children's feelings about themselves and other features of their lives.

(cont.)

The Teacher Interview

Although it is not necessarily conducted on the same day, the teacher interview is an essential part of your child's evaluation. Next to parents, few other adults will have spent more time with your child than his/her teachers, particularly if the child is of elementary school age. The opinions the teachers hold of the children are a critical part of the evaluation of any child and will be obtained by our professionals in most cases. In all but the most unusual circumstances, you should consent to this exchange of information, as it is in the best interest of your child's evaluation. This interview will likely be done by telephone.

The teachers most likely will be questioned about your child's current academic and behavioral problems. Relations with classmates also may be covered during this discussion. How your child acts in various school situations, especially where work has to be done, will likely be covered. We also like to ask teachers about situations that involve limited or no supervision, such as during recess, lunch, or special assemblies; while in hallways or bathrooms; or on the bus. The professional should also find out what the teachers are currently doing to manage the child's problems. Your child's performance in each academic subject should be briefly discussed. The professional may ask if your child has received a multidisciplinary team evaluation as part of the child's rights under state laws. If not, the professional may question the teacher as to whether one should be initiated in case special educational resources are going to be needed to help your child.

SUMMARY

Interviews with you and your child and contact with your child's teachers form an indispensable part of our evaluation of your child. These interviews provide a wealth of information useful to making a diagnosis and planning treatments for your child that simply cannot be obtained by any other means. Throughout these interviews, sufficient time must be taken by the professional to explore the necessary topics with each person to obtain as thorough a picture of your child as needed. A 20-minute initial interview will simply not suffice! The average length of time devoted to interviewing alone is often 1–2 hours, not including any psychological testing of the child. It will also be important for the professional to obtain parent and teacher behavior rating scales of your child's behavior. Some children will also require academic or psychological testing to rule out other developmental or learning disabilities, but these will not be done on the day of your evaluation. If they are needed, you will be told by your professional as to why testing is needed and where it can be obtained.

We hope you have found this pamphlet useful in preparing for your child's evaluation with our professional staff.

CLINICAL INTERVIEW—PARENT REPORT FORM (FORM 9)

Child's name_____ **Informant**_____

Informant's relationship to child: [*Circle one*]   Mother   Father   Other:_____

Record/chart #_____ Interviewer_____ Date_____

Child's date of birth_____ Age: Years_____ Months_____

Referral source_____ (e.g., school, physician, etc.)

Does referring person wish a copy of the report from this evaluation?   Yes   No

Clinical Diagnoses: [*To be filled in after evaluation is completed*]

1._____ 2._____ 3._____

Clinical Recommendations: [*To be briefly listed after evaluation is completed*]

1. _____
2. _____
3. _____
4. _____
5. _____
6. _____
7. _____
8. _____
9. _____
10. _____

LEGAL DISCLOSURES

[*Interviewer: At the start of the interview, be certain to review any necessary legal disclosures pertinent to your state, county, or other geographic region. For instance, in Massachusetts, we advise parents of the following four issues:*

1. *Any disclosure of information that indicates a suspicion of child abuse must be reported to state authorities (Department of Social Services).*

(cont.)

2. Any disclosure of threats of harm to oneself, as in a specific suicide threat, will result in immediate referral to an emergency mental health unit.
3. Any disclosure of specific threats to specific individuals will result in notification of those individuals concerning the threat.
4. Although the mental health records are confidential, they may be subpoenaed by a judge's order and must be provided to the court if so ordered.

Take time now to cover any such issues with the family before proceeding to the remainder of this interview.]

FAMILY COMPOSITION

Is this child: _____Your biological child _____Adopted _____Foster child

With which parent does the child live? _____Both _____Mother only _____Father only

_____Neither parent; child lives with _____Grandparent _____In foster care

Do you have legal custody of this child?   Yes   No   [*Interviewer: If No, determine whether or not it is legally advisable or permissible to proceed with this evaluation.*]

Does any other adult live in the home?   Yes   No   If so, who is it?_____

How many children are in the family?_____ How many are still at home?_____

PARENTAL CONCERNS ABOUT CHILD—REASONS FOR EVALUATION

What are you most concerned about regarding your child that led you to request this evaluation? [*Organize parent's responses under major headings below. Query parents about (1) the specific details of each concern, (2) when it began, (3) how often it occurs or how severe it is, and (4) what they have tried to do so far to deal with it.*]

Home behavior management problems:

Home emotional reaction problems:

(cont.)

Developmental delays: [*If present, consider reviewing with parents the diagnostic criteria for Mental Retardation or other specific developmental disorders such as learning disorders.*]

School behavior management problems:

School work performance or learning problems:

School emotional reaction problems:

Social interaction problems with peers:

Behavior in the community (outside of home and school):

Other concerns:

Why have you decided to seek this evaluation of your child at this time?

(cont.)

What type of assistance or treatment recommendations do you hope to receive from this evaluation?

Now that you have told me what your main concerns about your child are that bring you here today and what you hope to gain from the evaluation, I need to go over a number of different topics with you about your child. This needs to be done to be sure that I get as comprehensive a picture of your child's psychological adjustment as possible. I am going to ask you about a number of important developmental areas for any child. You should tell me if you have noticed anything unusual, abnormal, atypical, or even bizarre about your child's functioning in any of these areas. Let's begin with your child's:

Sensory development (impairments in vision, hearing, sense of touch or smell; abnormal reactions to sensory stimulation; hallucinations, etc.):

Motor development (coordination, gait, balance, posture, movements, gestures, tics, nervous habits or mannerisms, etc.):

Language development (delays, comprehension problems, speech difficulties):

Emotional development (overreactions, mood swings, extreme or unpredictable moods, peculiar or odd emotions, unusual fears or anxieties, etc.):

Thinking (odd ideas, bizarre preoccupations or fixations, unusual fantasies, speaks in incomplete or incoherent thoughts, delusions):

(cont.)

Social behavior (aggressive, rejected, bullies others, withdrawn, shy, anxious around others, mute when with others, aloof from others or shows no desire for friends/playmates, etc.):

Intelligence/academic skills (delays in general mental development; problems with memory; or specific delays in reading, math, spelling, handwriting, or other academic skill areas):

REVIEW OF DSM-IV CHILDHOOD DISORDERS

Now I need to ask you about a number of very specific questions about a variety of behavioral, social, or emotional problems that children sometimes have difficulties with. As I ask you about these things, keep in mind that some of these things are not bad or abnormal and may be seen sometimes in healthy, normal children. I want you to tell me if your child does any of these things to a degree that you consider to be inappropriate for someone of his/her age and sex.

[*Interviewer: If this child is a member of a minority group in this country or used to reside in a foreign country, be sure to follow up any answer by the parent that endorses a symptom as present with the following question: "Yes, but do you consider this to be a problem or to be inappropriate for a child of your ethnic or cultural group?"*]

Oppositional Defiant Disorder

[*Interviewer: Diagnosis requires four or more symptoms. Symptoms must be inappropriate for child's age; have lasted at least the past 6 months; and must be producing clear evidence of clinically significant impairment in social, academic, or occupational functioning.*]

I am now going to ask you some specific questions about your child's behavior during the past 6 months. For each of the behaviors I ask you about, please tell me if your child shows that behavior to a degree that is inappropriate compared to other children of your child's age.

A. Oppositional Defiant List [*Enter 1 if present, 0 if absent, and ? if unknown.*]

   During the past 6 months, did your child show any of the following:

   1. Often loses temper   ____
   2. Often argues with adults   ____

(cont.)

Note. The questions in the remainder of this form are adapted from the diagnostic criteria of the DSM-IV (American Psychiatric Association, 1994). Copyright 1994 by the American Psychiatric Association. Adapted by permission.

3. Often actively defies or refuses to comply with adults' requests or rules   ____
4. Often deliberately annoys people   ____
5. Often blames others for his/her own mistakes or misbehavior   ____
6. Is often touchy or easily annoyed by others   ____
7. Is often angry or resentful   ____
8. Is often spiteful or vindictive   ____

B. Have these behaviors existed for at least the past 6 months?   ____

[*Enter 1 if present, 0 if absent, and ? if unknown.*]

C. At what age did these behaviors first cause problems for your child? ____ (yrs.)

D. Have these behaviors created problems or impairment for your child in either of the following areas? [*Enter 1 if present, 0 if absent, and ? if unknown.*]

Social relations with others ____ Academic performance ____

E. Exclusion Criteria: [*Interviewer: Enter 1 if symptoms occur only during a Psychotic Disorder or Mood Disorder or if criteria are met for Conduct Disorder. Enter 0 if not, ? if unknown.*] ____

Diagnostic Code

Requirements for diagnosis:

Does section A total 4 or more?   ____
Does section B total 1?   ____
Does section D total 1 or more?   ____
Does section E total 0?   ____

[*Check here if all requirements are met*]

☐ ODD (313.81)

Conduct Disorder

[*Interviewer: Diagnosis requires three or more symptoms during previous 12 months and at least one during the past 6 months; the symptoms must presently be causing impairment in social or academic functioning.*]

Now I want to ask you about some other things your child may have done. For these behaviors, I want you to think about the past 12 months and tell me whether any of these have occurred during that time.

A. Conduct Disorder List [*Enter 1 if present, 0 if absent, and ? if unknown.*]

During the past 12 months, did your child do any of the following:

1. Often bullies, threatens, or intimidates others   ____
2. Often initiates physical fights   ____

(cont.)

3. Has used a weapon that can cause serious physical harm to others (e.g., a bat, brick, broken bottle, knife, or gun)   ____
4. Has been physically cruel to people   ____
5. Has been physically cruel to animals   ____
6. Has stolen while confronting a victim (e.g., mugging, purse snatching, extortion, armed robbery)   ____
7. Has forced someone into sexual activity   ____
8. Has deliberately engaged in fire setting with the intention of causing serious damage   ____
9. Has deliberately destroyed others' property (other than by fire setting)   ____
10. Has broken into someone else's house, building, or car   ____
11. Often lies to obtain goods or favors or to avoid obligations (i.e., "cons" others)   ____
12. Has stolen items of nontrivial value without confronting a victim (e.g., shoplifting, but without breaking and entering; forgery)   ____
13. Often stays out at night despite parental prohibitions   ____
    If so, at what age did this begin? ____ (yrs.)
    [Interviewer: Must begin before age 13 years to be counted as a symptom.]
14. Has run away from home overnight at least twice while living in parent's home, foster care, or group home   ____
    If so, how many times?   ____
    [Interviewer: Count as a symptom if it occurred once without child returning for a lengthy period.]
15. Is often truant from school   ____
    If so, at what age did he/she begin doing this? ____ (yrs.)
    [Interviewer: Must begin before age 13 years to be counted as a symptom.]

B. Have three of these behaviors occurred during the past 12 months?   ____

   [Enter 1 if present, 0 if absent, and ? if unknown.]

C. Has at least one of these behaviors occurred during the past 6 months?   ____

   [Enter 1 if present, 0 if absent, and ? if unknown.]

D. Did any of these behaviors occur prior to age 10 years?   ____

   [Enter 1 if present, 0 if absent, and ? if unknown.]

E. Have these behaviors created problems or impairment for your child in either of the following areas? [Enter 1 if present, 0 if absent, and ? if unknown.]

   Social relations with others ____ Academic performance ____

F. Exclusion Criteria: [Interviewer: Enter 1 if the child is 18 years of age or older and criteria are met for Antisocial Personality Disorder. Enter 0 if not, ? if unknown.]   ____

(cont.)

Diagnostic Code

Requirements for diagnosis:

Does section A total 3 or more? ____
Does section B total 1? ____
Does section C total 1? ____
Does section E total 1 or more? ____
Does section F total 0? ____

[*Check one subtype if all requirements are met*]

☐ CD, Childhood-Onset Type (312.8) [*Onset of at least one symptom prior to age 10 years*]
☐ CD, Adolescent-Onset Type (312.8) [*Absence of any symptoms prior to age 10 years*]

Severity: [*Check appropriate severity level*]

☐ Mild [*Few, if any, conduct problems in excess of those required to make the diagnosis and conduct problems cause only minor harm to others.*]
☐ Moderate [*Number of conduct problems and effect on others is intermediate between "mild" and "severe."*]
☐ Severe [*Many conduct problems have occurred in excess of those required to make the diagnosis or conduct problems cause considerable harm to others.*]

Disruptive Behavior Disorder, NOS

[*Interviewer: This category is for disruptive disorders characterized by conduct or oppositional defiant behaviors that do not meet criteria for CD or ODD but that produce clinically significant impairment.*]

Disruptive Behavior Disorder, NOS (312.9)

Attention-Deficit/Hyperactivity Disorder

[*Interviewer: Diagnosis requires six Inattention symptoms and/or six Hyperactive–Impulsive symptoms. Symptoms must also be inappropriate for child's age, have lasted at least the past 6 months, and have caused some impairment prior to age 7 years; presently must be causing impairment in two situations (home, school, or work functioning); and must be producing clear evidence of clinically significant impairment in social or academic functioning.*]

Let me ask you about some other behaviors that your child may have shown during the past 6 months. Again, for each of the behaviors I ask you about, please tell me if your child shows that behavior to a degree that is inappropriate compared to other children of your child's age.

A. Inattention List [*Enter 1 if present, 0 if absent, and ? if unknown.*]

During the past 6 months, did your child show any of the following:

1. Often fails to give close attention to details or makes careless mistakes in schoolwork, work, or other activities ____

(*cont.*)

    2. Often has difficulty sustaining attention in tasks or play activities   ____

    3. Often does not seem to listen when spoken to directly   ____

    4. Often does not follow through on instructions and fails to finish schoolwork, chores, or duties at work [*Interviewer: Inquire to be sure this is not due solely to oppositional behavior or failure to understand instructions.*]   ____

    5. Often has difficulty organizing tasks and activities   ____

    6. Often avoids, dislikes, or is reluctant to engage in tasks that require sustained mental effort (such as schoolwork or homework)   ____

    7. Often loses things necessary for tasks or activities (e.g., toys, school assignments, pencils, books, or tools)   ____

    8. Is often easily distracted by extraneous stimuli   ____

    9. Is often forgetful in daily activities   ____

B. Hyperactive–Impulsive List [*Enter 1 if present, 0 if absent, and ? if unknown.*]

During the past 6 months, did your child show any of the following:

    1. Often fidgets with hands or feet or squirms in his/her seat   ____

    2. Often leaves his/her seat in the classroom or in other situations in which remaining seated is expected   ____

    3. Often runs about or climbs excessively in situations in which it is inappropriate to do so [*Interviewer: For adolescents, this may be limited to subjective feelings of restlessness.*]   ____

    4. Often has difficulty playing or engaging in leisure activities quietly   ____

    5. Is often "on the go" or often acts as if "driven by a motor"   ____

    6. Often talks excessively   ____

    7. Often blurts out answers before questions have been completed   ____

    8. Often has difficulty awaiting his/her turn   ____

    9. Often interrupts or intrudes on others (e.g., butts into conversations or games)   ____

C. Have these behaviors existed for at least the past 6 months?   ____

[*Enter 1 if present, 0 if absent, and ? if unknown.*]

D. At what age did these behaviors first cause problems for your child? [*Interviewer: Onset by age 13 is acceptable, although DSM-IV stipulates age 7.*] ____ (yrs.)

E. During the past 6 months, have these behaviors caused problems for this child in any of these situations? [*Enter 1 if present, 0 if absent, and ? if unknown.*]

At home ____ In school ____ At daycare or babysitters ____

In community activities (clubs, sports, scouts, etc.) ____

F. Have these behaviors created problems or impairment for your child in any of the following areas? [*Enter 1 if present, 0 if absent, and ? if unknown.*]

Social relations with others ____ Academic performance ____

(cont.)

G. Exclusion Criteria: [*Interviewer: Enter 1 if symptoms occur only during a Pervasive Developmental Disorder or Psychotic Disorder or are better accounted for by another mental disorder, such as a Mood, Anxiety, Dissociative, or Personality Disorder. Enter 0 if not, ? if unknown.*] ____

Diagnostic Code

Requirements for diagnosis:

Does section A total 6 or more, or does section B total 6 or more? ____
Does section C total 1? ____
Does section E total 2 or more? ____
Does section F total 1 or more? ____
Does section G total 0? ____

[*Check one subtype if all requirements are met*]

☐ ADHD, Combined Type (314.01) [*Meets criteria for both Inattention and Hyperactive–Impulsive lists*]
☐ ADHD, Predominantly Inattentive Type (314.00) [*Meets criteria only for Inattention items*]
☐ ADHD, Predominantly Hyperactive–Impulsive Type (314.01) [*Meets criteria only for Hyperactive–Impulsive items*]
☐ ADHD, NOS (Not Otherwise Specified) (314.9) [*For disorders with prominent symptoms that do not meet full criteria for any subtype of ADHD*]

For individuals (especially adolescents and adults) who currently have symptoms that no longer meet full criteria, specify "In Partial Remission": _____

ANXIETY AND MOOD DISORDERS

Now I would like to ask you some questions about your child's emotions in general and his/her emotional reactions to some specific situations. I'll begin by asking you about any specific fears that your child may have. Then I will ask you about his/her general mood or emotional condition throughout much of the day. Let's start with some specific fears that your child may have.

Specific Phobia

[*Interviewer: Diagnosis requires that each criteria A–F below be met.*]

A. Does your child show a marked and persistent fear that is excessive or unreasonable in response to the presence of or the anticipation of a specific object or situation? For instance, in response to or anticipation of certain animals, heights, being in the dark, thunderstorms or lightning, flying, receiving an injection, seeing blood, or any other things or situations? ____

[*Enter 1 if present, 0 if absent, and ? if unknown.*]

(cont.)

Diagnostic Code

　　Requirements for diagnosis:

　　　　Does section A total 2?　　　　　　　　　　 ____
　　　　Does each section B through F total 1 or more? ____
　　　　Does section G total 0?　　　　　　　　　　 ____

　　[*Check here if all requirements are met*]

　　☐ Social Phobia (300.23)
　　　　Specify if Generalized (fear includes most social situations): _____

Separation Anxiety Disorder

[*Interviewer: Diagnosis requires that at least three symptoms be present (see A below) for at least 4 weeks. The symptoms must have developed before age 18 years and must produce clinically significant distress or impairment in social, academic, or other important areas of functioning, and other disorders must be excluded as indicated below.*]

A. Separation Anxiety Disorder Symptom List:

　　Now let's talk about how your child reacts emotionally when he/she must be away from you or when he/she must leave home for activities in the community. Does your child show any of the following? [*Enter 1 if present, 0 if absent, and ? if unknown.*]

　　1. Recurrent, excessive distress when separation from home, or from a parent or major attachment figures, occurs or is anticipated ____

　　2. Persistent and excessive worry about losing a parent or major attachment figure or about possible harm occurring to such a figure ____

　　3. Persistent and excessive worry that an unexpected or untoward event will lead him/her to become separated from a parent or major attachment figure (e.g., getting lost or being kidnapped) ____

　　4. Persistent reluctance or refusal to go to school or elsewhere because of fear of separation ____

　　5. Persistent and excessive fear or reluctance to be alone, or without a parent or major attachment figure at home, or without such a parent or caregiver when in other settings ____

　　6. Persistent reluctance or refusal to go to sleep without being near a major attachment figure or to sleep away from home ____

　　7. Repeated nightmares involving the theme or topic of separation from a parent or other caregiver ____

　　8. Repeated complaints of physical symptoms, such as headaches, stomachaches, nausea, or vomiting, when separation from a parent or major attachment figure occurs or is anticipated ____

　　[*Interviewer: If three or more symptoms were endorsed, proceed with remaining criteria; otherwise, skip to next disorder. If any of the remaining criteria below are not met, skip to the next disorder.*]

(cont.)

B. Have these fears existed for at least 4 weeks? ____
[*Enter 1 if present, 0 if absent, and ? if unknown.*]

C. At what age did these behaviors first cause problems for your child? ____ (yrs.)
[*Interviewer: Symptoms must have developed before age 18 years.*]

D. Have these worries created distress for your child or impairment in any of the following areas?
[*Enter 1 if present, 0 if absent, and ? if unknown.*]

Social relations with others ____ Academic performance ____

Any other areas of functioning ____

E. Exclusion Criteria: [*Interviewer: Enter 1 if symptoms occur only during a Pervasive Developmental Disorder, Schizophrenia, or other Psychotic Disorder, or are not better accounted for by Panic Disorder. Enter 0 if not, ? if unknown.*] ____

Diagnostic Code

Requirements for diagnosis:

Does section A total 3 or more? ____
Does section B total 1? ____
Does section C show 17 years or less? ____
Does section D total 1 or more? ____
Does section E total 0? ____

[*Check here if all requirements are met.*]

☐ Separation Anxiety Disorder (309.21)
Specify if Early Onset (before age 6 years): _____

Generalized Anxiety Disorder

[*Interviewer: Diagnosis requires that criteria A and B be met; at least one symptom in criterion C be present for at least 6 months on more days than not; that symptoms produce clinically significant distress or impairment in social, academic, or other important areas of functioning; and that other disorders be excluded as indicated below.*]

Now let's talk about whether your child tends to be generally anxious or to worry a lot compared to other children of his/her age group.

A. [*Enter 1 if present, 0 if absent, and ? if unknown.*]
  1. Does your child show excessive anxiety and worry about a number of events or activities, such as work activities, school performance, or any other situations? ____
  2. Has this anxiety or worry occurred on more days than not for at least the last 6 months? ____

(cont.)

[Interviewer: If the questions in A above were endorsed, proceed with remaining criteria for this disorder; otherwise, skip to next disorder. If any of the remaining criteria below are not met, skip to the next disorder.]

B. Does your child find it difficult to control his/her worry? _____

C. Generalized Anxiety Disorder Symptom List:

Has your child's anxiety or worry been associated with any of the following behaviors for more days than not over the past 6 months? *[Enter 1 if present, 0 if absent, and ? if unknown.]*

[Interviewer: Only one condition needs to be present for this criterion to be met.]

1. Restlessness or feeling keyed up or on edge _____
2. Being easily fatigued or tired _____
3. Difficulty concentrating or mind going blank _____
4. Irritability _____
5. Muscle tension _____
6. Sleep disturbance or difficulties falling asleep, staying asleep, or restless and unsatisfying sleep _____

D. Have these worries created distress for your child or impairment in any of the following areas? *[Enter 1 if present, 0 if absent, and ? if unknown.]*

Social relations with others _____ Academic performance _____

Any other areas of functioning _____

E. Exclusion Criteria: *[Interviewer: Enter 1 if the anxiety or worry are confined to features of another mental disorder, such as being worried about having a panic attack (Panic Disorder), being embarrassed in public (Social Phobia), being contaminated (Obsessive–Compulsive Disorder), being away from home or major attachment figures (Separation Anxiety Disorder), having multiple physical complaints (Somatization Disorder), or having a serious illness (Hypochondriasis); or if the anxiety is associated with Posttraumatic Stress Disorder. Also, enter 1 if the disturbance is due to the direct physiological effects of a substance (e.g., drug abuse, medication) or a general medical condition (e.g., hyperthyroidism) or occurs exclusively during a Mood Disorder, a Psychotic Disorder, or a Pervasive Developmental Disorder. Enter 0 if not, ? if unknown.]* _____

Diagnostic Code

Requirements for diagnosis:

Does section A total 2? _____
Does section B total 1? _____
Does section C total 1 or more? _____
Does section D total 1 or more? _____
Does section E total 0? _____

[Check here if all requirements are met]

☐ Generalized Anxiety Disorder (300.02)

(cont.)

Dysthymic Disorder

[*Interviewer: Diagnosis requires that depressed mood exist for most of the day, for more days than not, for at least 1 year; that at least two symptoms from B exist; that the child has never been without the symptoms in A and B below for 2 consecutive months during the 1 year of the disturbance; that all exclusionary criteria are met; and that the symptoms cause clinically significant distress or impairment in social, academic, or other important areas of functioning.*]

I would like to speak with you now about your child's mood for most of the time.

A. [*Enter 1 if present, 0 if absent, and ? if unknown.*] Does your child show depressed mood or irritability for most of the day, by either his/her own report or your own observations of your child? ____

   Has this depressed mood occurred more days than not for at least the past 12 months? ____

   [*Interviewer: If the two questions in A above were endorsed, proceed with remaining criteria for this disorder; otherwise, skip to next disorder. If any of the remaining criteria are not met, skip to the next disorder.*]

B. Does your child show any of the following difficulties while he/she is depressed: [*Enter 1 if present, 0 if absent, and ? if unknown.*]

   1. Poor appetite or overeating ____
   2. Insomnia (trouble falling asleep) or hypersomnia (excessive sleeping) ____
   3. Low energy or fatigue ____
   4. Low self-esteem ____
   5. Poor concentration or difficulty making decisions ____
   6. Feelings of hopelessness ____

C. During the 12 months or more that your child has shown this depressed mood, has he/she ever been without this depressed mood or the other difficulties you mentioned for at least 2 consecutive months? ____

   [*Enter 0 if the child has had a 2-month remission, 1 if he/she has not had any remission of symptoms for at least 2 months, and ? if unknown.*]

D. Has this depressed mood created distress for your child or impairment in any of the following areas? [*Enter 1 if present, 0 if absent, and ? if unknown.*]

   Social relations with others ____ Academic performance ____

   Any other areas of functioning ____

E. Exclusion Criteria: [*Interviewer: Enter 1 if the child meets criteria for Major Depressive Episode during the year or more of his/her mood disorder or if the disorder is better accounted for by Major Depressive Disorder. Also, enter 1 if there has ever been a manic episode, mixed manic–depressive episode, or hypomanic episode; or if criteria for Cyclothymic Disorder apply. Enter 1 if the disorder described above occurs exclusively during the course of a chronic Psychotic Disorder Schizophrenia or Delusional Disorder or is the result of the direct physiological effects of a substance or a general medical condition. Enter 0 if not, ? if unknown.*] ____

(cont.)

Diagnostic Code

Requirements for diagnosis:

Does section A total 2? ——
Does section B total 2 or more? ——
Does section C total 1? ——
Does section D total 1 or more? ——
Does section E total 0? ——

[*Check here if all requirements are met*]

☐ Dysthymic Disorder (300.4)

Major Depressive Disorder

[*Interviewer: Diagnosis requires that at least five or more of the symptoms listed in A below have been present for a 2-week period; that this represents a change from previous functioning; that at least one of the symptoms is depressed mood or loss of interest or pleasure; that the symptoms create clinically significant distress or impairment in social, academic, or other important areas of functioning; and that all exclusion criteria are met.*]

A. Major Depressive Disorder Symptom List:

Let's continue to talk about your child's mood or emotional adjustment. Has your child developed any of the following for at least a 2-week period of time? [*Enter 1 if present, 0 if absent, and ? if unknown.*]

1. Depressed or irritable mood most of the day nearly every day for at least 2 weeks ——
(This can be by the child's own report or by the parents' or others' observations.)

2. Markedly diminished interest or pleasure in all or almost all activities most of the day, nearly every day for at least 2 weeks ——
(This can be by the child's own report or by the parents' or others' observations.)
[*Interviewer: If either 1 or 2 was endorsed, proceed with remaining criteria; otherwise, skip to the next disorder.*]

3. Significant weight loss, when not dieting ——
Significant weight gain ——
Decrease or increase in appetite nearly every day ——
Failed to meet expected weight gains ——

4. Insomnia (trouble falling asleep) or hypersomnia (excessive sleep) nearly every day ——

5. Agitated or excessive movement nearly every day ——
(Must be supported by the parents' or others' observations)
Lethargic, sluggish, slow moving, or significantly reduced movement or activity nearly every day ——
(Must be supported by the parents' or others' observations)

(*cont.*)

6. Fatigue or loss of energy nearly every day   ____

7. Feelings of worthlessness or excessive or inappropriate guilt nearly every day   ____
   [*Interviewer: This should not be just self-reproach or guilt about being sick.*]

8. Diminished ability to think or concentrate, or indecisiveness, nearly every day   ____
   (Can be by child's self-report or parent's or others' observations.)

9. Recurrent thoughts of death   ____
   Recurrent thoughts of suicide without a specific plan   ____
   Suicide attempt or a specific plan for committing suicide   ____

[*Interviewer: If five or more of symptoms 1–9 were endorsed, proceed. If not, skip to the next disorder.*]

B. Have these symptoms of depression created distress for your child or impairment in any of the following areas? [*Enter 1 if present, 0 if absent, and ? if unknown.*]

   Social relations with others ____ Academic performance ____

   Any other areas of functioning ____

C. Exclusion Criteria: [*Interviewer: Enter 1 if the child meets criteria for Bipolar Disorder; if the symptoms are due to direct physiological effects of a substance or a general medical condition; if the symptoms are better accounted for by clinical Bereavement after the loss of a loved one or by Schizoaffective Disorder; if the symptoms are superimposed on Schizophrenia, Schizophreniform Disorder, Delusional Disorder, or Psychotic Disorder NOS; or if there has been a Manic Episode, a Mixed Episode, or a Hypomanic Episode. Enter 0 if not, ? if unknown.*]   ____

Diagnostic Code

   Requirements for diagnosis:

        Do questions 1 and 2 in section A total 1 or more?   ____
        Does section A total 5 or more?   ____
        Does section B total 1 or more?   ____
        Does section C total 0?   ____

   [*Check here if all requirements are met*]

   ☐ Major Depressive Disorder (296.xx)
   [*Code for single episode is 296.2x, recurrent episodes is 296.3x; see pp. 344–345 of DSM-IV for additional specifications about the disorder.*]

Depressive Disorder, NOS

[*Interviewer: Code this only where there is clinically significant depression with impairment, but where full criteria for Major Depressive Disorder, Dysthymic Disorder, Adjustment Disorder with Depressed Mood, or Adjustment Disorder with Mixed Anxiety and Depressed Mood are not met.*]

   ☐ Depressive Disorder, NOS (311)

(cont.)

Bipolar I Disorder: Manic Episode

[*Interviewer: Diagnosis requires that the child has had a distinct period of at least 1 week of abnormally and persistently elevated, expansive, or irritable mood, or any period of such mood that resulted in hospitalization; and has had at least three of the symptoms listed in B below (or four if mood was primarily irritable) to a significant degree. Also, the symptoms must create clinically significant impairment in social, academic, or other important areas of functioning; and exclusion criteria must be met.*]

I have some more questions to ask you about your child's moods or emotional adjustment.

A. Has your child ever experienced a period of time that lasted at least 1 week: [*Enter 1 if present, 0 if absent, and ? if unknown.*]

- Where his/her mood was unusually and persistently elevated; that is, he/she felt abnormally happy, giddy, joyous, or ecstatic well beyond normal feelings of happiness? ____
- Or, where his/her mood was abnormally and persistently expansive; that is, your child felt able to accomplish everything he/she decided to do, felt nearly superhuman in his/her ability to do anything he/she wished to do, or felt as if his/her abilities were without limits? ____
- Or, where his/her mood was abnormally and persistently irritable; that is, he/she was unusually touchy, too easily prone to anger or temper outbursts, too easily annoyed by events or by others, or abnormally cranky? ____

[*Interviewer: If any of the above three were endorsed, proceed with B; otherwise, skip to next disorder.*]

B. During the week or more that your child showed this abnormal and persistent mood, did you notice any of the following to be persistent and/or occurring to an abnormal or significant degree? [*Enter 1 if present, 0 if absent, and ? if unknown.*]

1. Had inflated self-esteem or felt grandiose about self well beyond what would be characteristic for his/her level of abilities ____
2. Showed a decreased need for sleep; for instance, he/she stated that he/she felt rested after only 3 hours of sleep ____
3. Was more talkative than usual or seemed to feel pressured to keep talking ____
4. Skipped from one idea to another and then another in speech as if his/her ideas were flying rapidly by ____
    Stated that he/she felt that his/her thoughts were racing or flying by at an abnormal rate of speed ____
5. Was distractible; that is, his/her attention was too easily drawn to unimportant or irrelevant events or things around him/her ____
6. Showed an increase in goal-directed activity; that is, he/she became unusually and persistently productive or directed more activity than normal toward the tasks he/she wanted to accomplish ____
    Seemed very agitated, overly active, or abnormally restless ____
7. Showed an excessive involvement in pleasurable activities that have a high likelihood of negative, harmful, or painful consequences ____

(cont.)

[*Interviewer: If three or more symptoms above were endorsed, proceed with remaining criteria; otherwise, skip to next disorder.*]

C. [*Enter 1 if present, 0 if absent, and ? if unknown.*]

1. Was this disturbance in your child's mood enough to cause severe impairment, disruption, or difficulties with social relationships, academic performance, or other important activities   ____

2. Or, did your child's abnormal mood lead to him/her being hospitalized to prevent harm to him/herself or others   ____

3. Or, did your child have hallucinations (explain) or bizarre ideas (psychotic thinking), or feel or act paranoid (as if others were intentionally out to harm him/her)   ____

[*Interviewer: If one or more of the criteria 1–3 is endorsed, proceed.*]

D. Exclusion Criteria: [*Interviewer: Enter 1 if the symptoms meet criteria for Mixed Manic–Depressive Episode or Schizoaffective Disorder, are the direct physiological effects of a substance or a general medical condition, or are superimposed on Schizophrenia, Schizophreniform Delusional Disorder, or Psychotic Disorder NOS. Enter 0 if not, ? if unknown. Also, if the child meets criteria for ADHD, enter 0 only if the child meets the criteria after excluding distractibility (5, above) and psychomotor agitation (second part of 6, above).*]   ____

Diagnostic Code

Requirements for diagnosis:

Does section A total 1 or more? ____
Does section B total 3 or more? ____
Does section C total 1 or more? ____
Does section D total 0? ____

[*Check here if all requirements are met*]

☐ Bipolar I Disorder: Manic Episode (296.xx)
[*Code 296.0x if single episode; 296.40 if multiple episodes and most recent was Manic Episode; 296.4x if multiple episodes and most recent was Hypomanic Episode.*]

Bipolar I Disorder: Mixed Episode

[*Interviewer: Code this disorder if criteria are met both for a Manic Episode and for a Major Depressive Episode nearly every day for at least 1 week; disturbance causes clinically significant impairment; and symptoms are not the result of a substance or a general medical condition.*]

☐ Bipolar I Disorder: Mixed Episode (_____)
[*Code 296.6x if most recent episode is mixed; 296.5x if most recent episode is depressed; 296.7 if most recent episode is unspecified.*]

(cont.)

Other Mental and Developmental Disorders:

[Enter 1 if present, 0 if absent, and ? if unknown.]

1. Does this child have any things about which he/she seems obsessed or can he/she not get his/her mind off of a particular topic? ____ *[If present, review diagnostic criteria for Obsessive–Compulsive Disorder in the DSM-IV.]*
2. Does this child have any unusual behaviors he/she must perform, such as dressing, bathing, mealtime, or counting rituals? ____ *[If present, review diagnostic criteria for Obsessive–Compulsive disorder in the DSM-IV.]*
3. Does this child demonstrate any nervous tics or other repetitive, abrupt nervous movements or vocal noises? ____ *[If present, review diagnostic criteria for Tic Disorders or Tourette's Disorder in the DSM-IV.]*
4. Has this child made comments or acted in such a way that he/she seemed to see things, hear things, or feel things on his/her skin that really did not exist (hallucinations)? ____ *[If present, review diagnostic criteria for Psychotic Disorders in the DSM-IV.]*
5. Has this child ever reported bizarre or very strange or peculiar ideas that seemed very unusual compared to other children (delusions)? ____ *[If present, review diagnostic criteria for Psychotic Disorders in the DSM-IV.[*

PARENT MANAGEMENT METHODS

Now let's move on and talk about how you have tried to manage your child's behavior, especially when it was a problem for you. When your child is disruptive or misbehaves, what steps are you likely to take to deal with the problem?

_____
_____
_____
_____
_____
_____
_____

If these methods do not work and the problem behavior continues, what are you likely to do then to cope with your child's misbehavior?

_____
_____
_____
_____
_____
_____
_____

(cont.)

CHILD'S EVALUATION AND TREATMENT HISTORY

Has your child ever been evaluated previously for developmental, behavioral, or learning problems? [*Circle one*]   Yes   No

If so, who provided the evaluation, what type of evaluation did the child have, and what were you told about your child regarding the results of any evaluations?

_____
_____
_____
_____
_____

Has your child ever received any psychiatric or psychological treatment? [*Circle one*]   Yes   No

If so, what type of treatment did he/she receive and how long did the treatment last?

_____
_____

Who provided this treatment to your child?_____

Has your child ever received any *medication* for his/her behavior or emotional problems? [*Circle one*]   Yes   No

If so, what type of medication did he/she take, at what dose, and for how long?

_____
_____

SCHOOL HISTORY

[*Interviewer: For each grade the child has been in, beginning with preschool, ask the parents the school the child attended and whether the child had any behavioral or learning problems that year, and if so, briefly note their nature below.*]

_____
_____
_____
_____
_____
_____
_____
_____
_____
_____

(cont.)

Has this child ever received any *special education services*? [*Circle one*]   Yes   No

If so, what types of services did he/she receive and in what grades?

_____

_____

_____

_____

CHILD'S PSYCHOLOGICAL AND SOCIAL STRENGTHS

I realize I have asked you a lot about any problems your child might be having. But it is also important that I know about your child's psychological and social strong points. Please tell me about any abilities your child seems to have or any activities at which he/she is particularly good. For instance, what hobbies and sports does your child enjoy and do well at, what are his/her best subjects in school, what sorts of games or social activities does he/she do well in? In other words, tell me what you consider to be your child's strongest or best points.

_____

_____

_____

_____

_____

FAMILY HISTORY

[*Interviewer: After reviewing the child's psychological and social strengths, review with the parent the family history of psychiatric and learning problems, using the following three forms. One form is for the maternal side of the family, the second for the paternal side, and the third for the siblings of the child being evaluated. Inform the parent(s) you are interviewing that it is important in understanding a child's behavioral problems to know whether other biological relatives of the child have had psychological, emotional, or developmental problems. Many such disorders run in families and may contribute genetically to the child's problems. Start with the maternal side of the family and review each of the mother's relatives, noting whether they have any of the disorders listed on the left side of the form. If so, place an X in that box of the matrix in the column representing that relative. Then do the same for the paternal relatives and the child's siblings.*]

Maternal Relatives

	Self	Mother	Father	Siblings Bro	Bro	Sis	Sis	Total
Problems with aggressiveness, defiance, and oppositional behavior as a child								
Problems with attention, activity, and impulse control as a child								

(cont.)

	Self	Mother	Father	Siblings Bro	Bro	Sis	Sis	Total
Learning disabilities								
Failed to graduate from high school								
Mental retardation								
Psychosis or schizophrenia								
Depression for more than 2 weeks								
Anxiety disorder that impaired adjustment								
Tics or Tourette's								
Alcohol abuse								
Substance abuse								
Antisocial behavior (assaults, thefts, etc.)								
Arrests								
Physical abuse								
Sexual abuse								

Paternal Relatives

	Self	Mother	Father	Siblings Bro	Bro	Sis	Sis	Total
Problems with aggressiveness, defiance, and oppositional behavior as a child								
Problems with attention, activity, and impulse control as a child								
Learning disabilities								
Failed to graduate from high school								
Mental retardation								
Psychosis or schizophrenia								
Depression for more than 2 weeks								
Anxiety disorder that impaired adjustment								
Tics or Tourette's								
Alcohol abuse								
Substance abuse								

(cont.)

	Self	Mother	Father	Siblings Bro	Bro	Sis	Sis	Total
Antisocial behavior (assaults, thefts, etc.)								
Arrests								
Physical abuse								
Sexual abuse								

Siblings

	Brother	Brother	Sister	Sister	Total
Problems with aggressiveness, defiance, and oppositional behavior as a child					
Problems with attention, activity, and impulse control as a child					
Learning disabilities					
Failed to graduate from high school					
Mental retardation					
Psychosis or schizophrenia					
Depression for more than 2 weeks					
Anxiety disorder that impaired adjustment					
Tics or Tourette's					
Alcohol abuse					
Substance abuse					
Antisocial behavior (assaults, thefts, etc.)					
Arrests					
Physical abuse					
Sexual abuse					

ADULT BEHAVIOR RATING SCALE—SELF-REPORT OF CURRENT BEHAVIOR
(FORM 10)

Your name _____ **Age** _____ **Date** _____

Instructions: Circle the number that *best describes* your behavior over the past 6 months.

	Never or rarely	Sometimes	Often	Very often
1. Fail to give close attention to details or make careless mistakes in job tasks or schoolwork	0	1	2	3
2. Have difficulty sustaining attention in tasks or leisure activities	0	1	2	3
3. Do not seem to listen when spoken to directly	0	1	2	3
4. Do not follow through on instructions and fail to finish work	0	1	2	3
5. Have difficulty organizing tasks and activities	0	1	2	3
6. Avoid tasks (e.g., job tasks, schoolwork) that require mental effort	0	1	2	3
7. Lose things necessary for tasks or activities	0	1	2	3
8. Easily distracted	0	1	2	3
9. Forgetful in daily activities	0	1	2	3
10. Fidget with hands or feet or squirm in seat	0	1	2	3
11. Leave seat in situations in which remaining seated is expected	0	1	2	3
12. Move about excessively in situations in which it is inappropriate; hyperactive; subjective feelings of restlessness	0	1	2	3
13. Have difficulty engaging in leisure activities quietly	0	1	2	3
14. "On the go" or act as if "driven by a motor"	0	1	2	3
15. Talk excessively	0	1	2	3
16. Blurt out answers before questions have been completed	0	1	2	3
17. Have difficulty awaiting turn	0	1	2	3
18. Interrupt or intrude on others	0	1	2	3
19. Lose temper	0	1	2	3
20. Argue with others	0	1	2	3
21. Actively defy or refuse to comply with requests or rules	0	1	2	3
22. Deliberately annoy people	0	1	2	3
23. Blame others for my own mistakes or misbehavior	0	1	2	3
24. Touchy or easily annoyed by others	0	1	2	3
25. Angry and resentful	0	1	2	3
26. Spiteful or vindictive	0	1	2	3

ADULT BEHAVIOR RATING SCALE—SELF-REPORT OF CHILDHOOD BEHAVIOR (FORM 11)

Your name _____ Age _____ Date _____

Instructions: Circle the number that *best describes* your behavior as a child, ages 5–12 years.

	Never or rarely	Sometimes	Often	Very often
1. Failed to give close attention to details or made careless mistakes in schoolwork	0	1	2	3
2. Had difficulty sustaining attention in tasks or play activities	0	1	2	3
3. Did not seem to listen when spoken to directly	0	1	2	3
4. Did not follow through on instructions and failed to finish work	0	1	2	3
5. Had difficulty organizing tasks and activities	0	1	2	3
6. Avoided tasks (e.g., schoolwork, homework) that required mental effort	0	1	2	3
7. Lost things necessary for tasks or activities	0	1	2	3
8. Easily distracted	0	1	2	3
9. Forgetful in daily activities	0	1	2	3
10. Fidgeted with hands or feet or squirmed in seat	0	1	2	3
11. Left seat in classroom or in other situations in which remaining seated was expected	0	1	2	3
12. Ran about or climbed excessively in situations in which it was inappropriate; hyperactive	0	1	2	3
13. Had difficulty engaging in play activities quietly	0	1	2	3
14. "On the go" or acted as if "driven by a motor"	0	1	2	3
15. Talked excessively	0	1	2	3
16. Blurted out answers before questions had been completed	0	1	2	3
17. Had difficulty awaiting turn	0	1	2	3
18. Interrupted or intruded on others	0	1	2	3
19. Lost temper	0	1	2	3
20. Argued with adults	0	1	2	3
21. Actively defied or refused to comply with requests or rules	0	1	2	3
22. Deliberately annoyed people	0	1	2	3
23. Blamed others for my own mistakes or misbehavior	0	1	2	3
24. Touchy or easily annoyed by others	0	1	2	3
25. Angry and resentful	0	1	2	3
26. Spiteful or vindictive	0	1	2	3

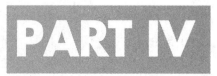

PART IV

Parent Handouts

The handouts provided in this section are to be used in conjunction with this training manual and the instructions associated with them provided in Part II of this manual. Permission is granted by the author and publisher for the purchaser of this manual to photocopy these handouts as necessary for use solely in the purchaser's professional practice and solely for the purpose of training parents in this program whose child is under the professional care of the purchaser (see the copyright page for details). These handouts also appear in a Spanish-language supplement available from the publisher.

Contents of Part IV

Parent Handout for Step 1: Profiles of Child and Parent Characteristics	219
Parent Handout for Step 1: Family Problems Inventory	220
Parent Handout for Step 2: Paying Attention to Your Child's Good Play Behavior	222
Parent Handout for Step 3: Paying Attention to Your Child's Compliance	225
Parent Handout for Step 3: Giving Effective Commands	227
Parent Handout for Step 3: Attending to Independent Play	228
Parent Handout for Step 4: The Home Poker Chip/Point System	230
Parent Handout for Step 5: Time Out!	233
Parent Handout for Step 7: Anticipating Problems—Managing Children in Public Places	237
Parent Handout for Step 8: Using a Daily School Behavior Report Card	240
Parent Handout for Step 9: Managing Future Behavior Problems	247

PARENT HANDOUT FOR STEP 1:
PROFILES OF CHILD AND PARENT CHARACTERISTICS

Child's name_____ **Age**_____

Name of parent completing form_____

Relationship to child:_____ Date_____

CHILD CHARACTERISTICS

Please list below any characteristics of your child that you believe may be contributing the child's behavioral difficulties:

Health problems:_____
Physical problems:_____
Developmental delays:_____
Problems with impulse control:_____
Problems with attention span:_____
Problems with activity level:_____
Social behavior problems:_____
Problems with sleeping or eating:_____
Toilet training problems:_____
Emotional problems, irritability:_____
Other problems:_____

PARENT CHARACTERISTICS

List below any problems of your own that you believe may contribute to difficulties you have in managing your child or children:

Health problems:_____
Physical problems:_____
Emotional problems:_____
Thinking problems:_____
Problems with:
    Attention span?_____ Activity level?_____
    Impulse control?_____ Moodiness?_____
    Eating?_____ Sleeping?_____
Other problems:_____

PARENT HANDOUT FOR STEP 1: FAMILY PROBLEMS INVENTORY

Child's name_____ Date_____

Name of parent completing this form_____

Instructions: Sometime during the next week, take some time to complete this questionnaire. You have been shown that one source of trouble that can contribute to child behavior problems is stress within the family. This questionnaire is designed to help you take inventory of possible stress events that may be occurring within your family. We think it is important that you "take stock" of these stressors and start to think about how you might begin to resolve them, if possible.

Listed below are common areas of stress within families. In the space provided below each, please write down any problems that you feel you or your family are having in these areas. Then next to each one, under the column marked "Proposed Solutions," list what you believe you can begin to do to help reduce these problems, if that is possible. Please be as honest as you can—your answers will be kept confidential.

Problem Areas	**Proposed Solutions**

1. Family health problems:

2. Marital problems:

3. Financial problems:

4. Behavior problems with other children in family:

(cont.)

5. Occupational/employment problems:

6. Problems with relatives/in-laws:

7. Problems with friends:

8. Other sources of stress (religion, conflict
   over recreational activities for family, drug
   or alcohol abuse, etc.):

Thank you for taking time to complete this inventory. Your therapist will review it and may decide to talk with you privately about some of these stressors. If you would like your therapist to help you with any of these problems or refer you to other people who may be able to assist you, please indicate that below by checking Yes or No and simply writing the number of the problem area(s) from above.

_____ Yes, I would like help with these areas (list numbers): _____
_____ No, I do not need help with these problem areas.

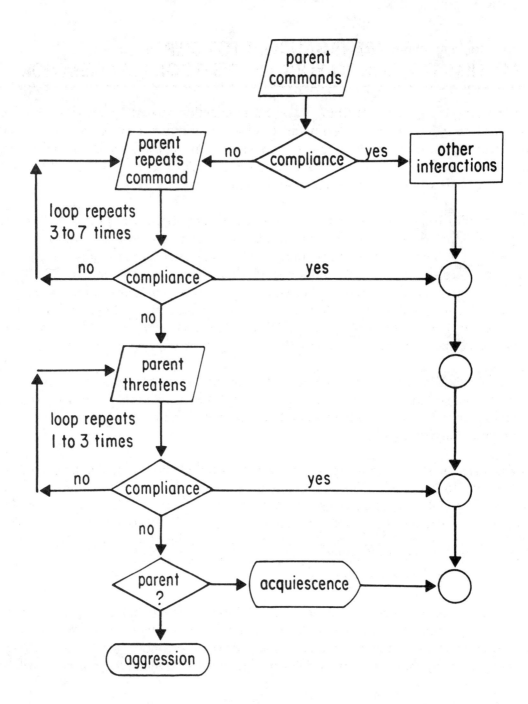

Diagram of Oppositional Defiant Interaction

PARENT HANDOUT FOR STEP 2:
PAYING ATTENTION TO YOUR CHILD'S GOOD PLAY BEHAVIOR

This step of the program involves learning how to pay attention to your child's desirable behavior when it happens during playtime. To learn this, it is first necessary to practice the skills of what we call "paying attention." Later, we will show you how to use these new "attending" skills to increase your child's compliance with commands and requests as well as other positive behavior. Paying attention to your child's play behavior involves the following:

1. If your child is below 9 years of age, select a time each day that is to become your "special time" with your child. This can be after other children are off to school in the morning if you have a preschool child, or after school or dinner if your child is of school age. You are to set aside 20 minutes each day at this time in order to practice this special playtime with your child. If your child is 9 years or older, you do not have to choose a standard time each day for this special time. Instead, find a time each day as it may arise when your child seems to be enjoying a play activity alone. Then, stop what you are doing and begin to join in the child's play, following the instructions below.

2. No other children are to be involved in this special playtime! If you have other children in your family, either have your spouse look after these children while you play with the problem child or choose a time when the other children are not likely to disturb your special time with this child.

3. If you have set up a standard special playtime each day, then when that time comes around simply say to your child, "It's now our special time to play together. What would you like to do?" The child is to choose the play activity, within reason. This should not be a time for watching television. Any other play activity is fine. If you have not set up a standard special playtime, then simply approach your child while he/she is playing alone and ask if you can join in. In either case, the parent is not to take control of the play or direct it—the child is to choose the play activity.

4. **Relax!!!** Casually watch what your child is doing for a few minutes, and then join in where it seems appropriate. Do not try to do this special playtime when you are upset, very busy, or planning to leave the house immediately for some errand or trip, as your mind will be preoccupied by these matters and the quality of your attention to your child will be quite poor.

5. After watching your child's play, begin to describe out loud what your child is doing. This is done to show your child that you find his/her play interesting. It is done something like the way a sportscaster might describe a baseball or football game over the radio. It should be somewhat exciting and action oriented, not dull and in a single tone of voice. In other

(cont.)

words, occasionally narrate your child's play. Young children really enjoy this. With older children, you should still comment about their play, but less so than with a young child.

6. **Ask no questions and give no commands!!!** This is critical. You are to avoid any questioning of the child where possible, as this is often unnecessary and certainly disruptive to your child's play. It is all right to ask a question to clarify how your child is playing if you are uncertain of what he/she is doing. Otherwise, avoid any questions. Also, give no commands or directions and do not try to teach the child anything during this play. This is your child's special time to relax and enjoy your company, not a time to teach or take over the child's play.

7. Occasionally, provide your child with positive statements of praise, approval, or positive feedback about what you like about his/her play. Be accurate and honest, not excessively flattering. For instance, "I like it when we play quietly like this," "I really enjoy our special time together," or "Look at how nicely you have made that . . ." are all positive, appropriate comments. If you need help thinking of these comments, see the last page of this handout for a list of ways to show approval to your child.

8. If your child begins to misbehave, simply turn away and look elsewhere for a few moments. If the misbehavior continues, then tell your child that the special playtime is over and leave the room. Tell your child you will play with him/her later when he/she can behave nicely. If the child becomes extremely disruptive, destructive, or abusive during play, discipline the child as you might normally do. Your therapist will teach you effective disciplining later in this program.

9. Each parent is to spend 20 minutes with the child in this special playtime. During the first week, try to do this every day or at least 5 times in a week. After the first week, try to have this special time at least 3 to 4 times per week. You should continue this special playtime indefinitely.

This program is easy to read, it is not easy to do!!! Many parents make mistakes during the first few playtimes, usually by giving too many commands and questions or not making enough positive comments to the child. Don't worry about making such mistakes. Just try harder the next time to improve your "attending" skills toward your child. You may want to spend this kind of special playtime with the other children in your family once you have improved your attending skills with the problem child.

SUGGESTIONS FOR GIVING POSITIVE FEEDBACK AND APPROVAL TO YOUR CHILD

Nonverbal Signs of Approval

Hug
Pat on the head or shoulder
Affectionate rubbing of hair
Placing arm around the child

(cont.)

Smiling
A light kiss
Giving a "thumbs-up" sign
A wink

Verbal Approval

"I like it when you. . . . "
"It's nice when you. . . . . "
"You sure are a big boy/girl for. . . . "
"That was terrific the way you. . . . "
"Great job!"
"Nice going!"
"Terrific!"
"Super!"
"Fantastic!"
"My, you sure act grown up when you. . . . "
"You know, 6 months ago you couldn't do that as well as you can now—you're really growing up fast!"
"Beautiful!"
"Wow!"
"Wait until I tell your mom/dad how nice you. . . . "
"What a nice thing to do. . . . "
"You did that all by yourself . . . , way to go."
"Just for behaving so well, you and I will. . . . "
"I am very proud of you when you. . . . "
"I always enjoy it when we . . . like this."

Note

1. Always be as immediate as possible with your approval. Don't wait!

2. Always be specific about what it is that you like.

3. Never give a back-handed compliment such as, "It's about time you cleaned your room. Why couldn't you do that before?!!"

PARENT HANDOUT FOR STEP 3:
PAYING ATTENTION TO YOUR CHILD'S COMPLIANCE

Although you first learned how to pay attention to your child's play during the special playtimes, you can now use these attending skills to provide approval to your child when he/she follows a command or request. When you give a command, give the child immediate feedback for how well he/she is doing. Don't just walk away, but stay and attend and comment positively.

1. As soon as you have given a command or request and your child begins to comply, praise the child for complying, using phrases such as the following:
   "I like it when you do as I ask."
   "It's nice when you do as I say."
   "Thanks for doing what Mom/Dad asked."
   "Look at how nicely (quickly, neatly, etc.) you are doing that. . . ."
   "Good boy/girl for. . . ."

Or use any other statement that specifically says you appreciate that he/she is doing what you asked. You can also use some of the methods of approval provided in your handout for Step 2.

2. Once you have attended to your child's compliance, if you must, you can leave for a few moments, but be sure to return frequently to praise your child's compliance.

3. If you should find your child has done a job or chore without being specifically told to do so, this is the time to provide especially positive praise to your child. You may even wish to provide your child with a small privilege for having done this, which will help your child remember and follow household rules without always being told to do so.

4. You should begin to use positive attention to your child for virtually every command you give him/her. In addition, this week you should choose two or three commands your child follows only inconsistently. You should make a special effort to praise and attend to your child whenever he/she begins to comply with these particular commands.

SETTING UP COMPLIANCE TRAINING PERIODS

Also, it is very important during the next 1–2 weeks that you take a few minutes and specifically train compliance in your child. You can do this very easily. Select a time when your child is not very busy and ask him/her to do very brief favors for you, such as, "Hand me a Kleenex (spoon, towel, magazine, etc.)," or "Can you reach that _____ for me?" We call these "fetch" commands, and they should involve only a very brief and simple effort from your child. Give about five or six of these in a row during these few minutes. As your child follows each one, be sure to provide specific praise for your child's compliance, such as, "I like it when you listen to me," or "It is really nice when you do as I ask," or "Thanks for doing what I asked."

Try to have several of these compliance training periods each day. Because the requests are very simple, most children (even behavior problem children) will do them. This provides an excellent opportunity to catch your child "being good" and to praise his/her compliance.

PARENT HANDOUT FOR STEP 3: GIVING EFFECTIVE COMMANDS

In our work with many behavior problem children, we have noticed that if parents simply change the way they give commands to their children, they can often achieve significant improvements in the child's compliance. When you are about to give a command or instruction to your child, be sure that you do the following:

1. *Make sure you mean it*! That is, never give a command that you do not intend to see followed up to its completion. When you make a request, plan on backing it up with appropriate consequences, both positive or negative, to show that you mean what you have said.

2. *Do not present the command as a question or favor.* State the command simply, directly, and in a businesslike tone of voice.

3. *Do not give too many commands at once.* Most children are able to follow only one or two instructions at a time. For now, try giving only one specific instruction at a time. If a task you want your child to do is complicated, then break it down into smaller steps and give only one step at a time.

4. *Make sure the child is paying attention to you.* Be sure that you have eye contact with the child. If necessary, gently turn the child's face toward yours to ensure that he/she is listening and watching when the command is given.

5. *Reduce all distractions before giving the command.* This is a very common mistake that parents make. Often, parents try to give instructions while a television, stereo, or video game is on. Parents cannot expect children to attend to them when something more entertaining is going on in the room. Either turn off these distractions yourself or tell the child to turn them off before giving the command.

6. *Ask the child to repeat the command.* This need not be done with each request, but can be done if you are not sure your child heard or understood the command. Also, for children with a short attention span, having them repeat the command appears to increase the likelihood they will follow it through.

7. *Make up chore cards.* If your child is old enough to have jobs to do about the home, then you may find it useful to make up a chore card for each job. This can simply be a 3 x 5 file card. Listed on it are the steps involved in correctly doing that chore. Then, when you want your child to do the chore, simply hand the child the card and state that this is what you want done. Of course, this is only for children who are old enough to read. These cards can greatly reduce the amount of arguing that occurs about whether a child has done a job or chore properly. You might also indicate on the card how much time it should take to be done and then set your kitchen timer for this time period so the child knows exactly when it is to be done.

If you follow these seven steps, you will find some improvement in your child's compliance with your requests. When used with the other methods your therapist will teach you, remarkable improvements can occur in how well your child listens and behaves.

PARENT HANDOUT FOR STEP 3: ATTENDING TO INDEPENDENT PLAY

Many parents of behavior problem children complain that they are unable to do things, such as talk on the phone, cook dinner, visit with a neighbor, and so forth, without the child interrupting what they are doing. The following steps were designed to help you teach your child to play independently of you when you must be busy with some other activity. It is a very simple procedure that requires you to pay attention and praise your child for staying away and not interrupting you. Many parents provide a lot of attention to a child who is interrupting them but almost no attention to the child when he/she stays away, plays independently, and does not interrupt. No wonder kids interrupt parents so much! To teach your child to stay away from you when you are busy, do the following:

1. When you are about to become occupied with some activity, such as a phone call, reading, fixing dinner, and so forth, give your child a direct command. This command should contain two instructions. One part of it tells the child what he/she is to be doing while you are busy, and the second part specifically tells them not to interrupt or bother you. For instance, you can say, "Mom has to talk on the telephone, so I want you to stay in this room and watch television and don't bother me." Remember, give the child something to do that he/she enjoys and tell him/her you do not want to be bothered while you are busy.

2. Then as you begin your activity, stop what you are doing after a moment, go to the child, and praise the child for staying away and not interrupting. Remind the child to stay with his/her assigned task and not to bother you. Return to what you were doing.

3. Then wait a few moments longer before returning to the child and again praising him/her for not bothering you. Return to your activity, wait a little longer, and again praise the child.

4. Over time, what you are trying to do is gradually to reduce how often you praise the child for not bothering you while you increase the length of time you can stay at your own task. Initially, you will have to interrupt what you are doing and go praise the child very frequently, say every 30 seconds to 2 minutes. After a few times like this, wait 3 minutes before praising the child. Then wait 5 minutes before praising the child. Each time, you return to what you are working on for a slightly longer period of time before going back to praise the child.

5. If it sounds like your child is about to leave what he/she was doing and come to bother you, immediately stop what you are doing, go to the child, praise him/her for not interrupting you, and redirect him/her to stay with the task you gave him/her. The task you give a child should *not* be a chore, but some interesting activity such as coloring, playing with a toy, watching television, cutting out pictures, and so forth.

6. By gradually decreasing how often you praise the child, you will be able to stay with your own task for longer and longer time periods while your child does not interrupt you. As

(cont.)

From *Defiant Children*. Copyright 1997 by The Guilford Press. Permission to photocopy this form is granted to purchasers of *Defiant Children* for personal use only (see copyright page for details).

soon as you finish what you are doing, go and provide special praise to your child for letting you complete your task. You may even periodically give your child a small privilege or reward for having left you alone while you worked on your project.

Here are some of the activities that parents normally do during which you should try this method to keep your child from bothering you:

Preparing a meal	Talking on the telephone
Talking to an adult	Reading or watching TV
Writing a letter	Visiting others' homes
Doing paperwork	Housecleaning
Talking at the dinner table	Accomplishing any special project

You should choose one or two of these types of activities with which you will practice this method this week. If you choose talking on the phone, you might want to have your spouse or a friend call you one or two times a day simply as a time to practice this method. That way, when important calls do come in, you have already gotten your child to begin to stay away from you so you can handle these calls with fewer interruptions.

PARENT HANDOUT FOR STEP 4: THE HOME POKER CHIP/POINT SYSTEM

When trying to manage a child with behavioral problems, it is common to find that praise is not enough to motivate the child to do chores, follow rules, or obey commands. As a result, it is necessary to set up a more powerful program to motivate the child. One such program that has been very successful with children is the Home Poker Chip Program (for children 4–7 years old) or the Home Point System (for children 8 years old and older). Your therapist will explain in detail how to set up such a program, but here are the steps to follow:

THE HOME POKER CHIP PROGRAM

1. Find or buy a set of plastic poker chips. If the child is 4 or 5 years old, then each chip, regardless of color, represents 1 chip. For 6- to 8-year-olds, the colors can represent different amounts: white = 1 chip, blue = 5 chips, and red = 10 chips. If you use the colors this way, take one of each color, tape it to a small piece of cardboard, and write on each chip how many chips it is worth. Post this card somewhere so your child can easily refer to it.

2. Sit down and explain to your child that you feel he/she has not been rewarded enough for doing nice things at home and you want to change all that. You want to set up a new reward program so your child can earn nice privileges and things for behaving properly. This sets a very positive tone to the program.

3. You and your child should make a nice bank in which he/she will keep the chips earned. A shoe box, coffee can (with a dull edge on the rim), a plastic jar, or some other container can serve as a bank. Have some fun decorating it with your child.

4. Now, you and your child should make up a list of the privileges you want your child to earn with the poker chips. These should include not just occasional special privileges (going to movies, roller skating, buying a toy) but also the everyday privileges your child takes for granted (television, video games, special toys already in the home, riding a bike, going over to a friend's home, etc.). Your therapist will explain what types of privileges you might include on this list. Be sure to have at least 10, and preferably 15, rewards on this list.

5. Now make up a second list that will contain the jobs and chores you often ask this child to perform. These can be typical household chores such as setting the table for a meal, clearing the table after a meal, cleaning a bedroom, making a bed, emptying wastebaskets, and so forth. Also put on the list things like getting dressed for school, getting ready for bed, washing and bathing, brushing teeth, or any other self-help tasks you give a child

(cont.)

that normally pose a problem for you. Your therapist can help you decide what types of jobs to put on this list for your child's age group and special problems.

6. Next, take each job or chore and decide how much you feel it is worth in chips. For 4- and 5-year-olds, assign from 1 to 3 chips for most tasks, and perhaps 5 for really big jobs. For 6- to 8-year-olds, use a range of 1 to 10 chips, and perhaps give a larger amount for big jobs. Remember, the harder the job, the more chips you will pay.

7. Take a moment and add up approximately how many chips you think your child will earn in a typical day if he/she does most of these jobs. Then, remembering this number, decide how many chips your child should have to pay for each of the rewards you listed. We generally suggest that two-thirds of the child's daily chips should be spent on his/her typical daily privileges. This allows the child to save about one-third of his/her chips every day toward the purchase of some of the very special rewards on the list. Don't worry about the exact numbers to use here. Just use your judgment as to how much each reward should cost, be fair, and charge more chips for the special rewards and less for the daily ones.

8. Be sure to tell your child that he/she will have a chance to earn "bonus" chips when he/she performs a chore in a nice, prompt, and pleasant manner. You will not give these bonus chips all the time, but should give them when your child has done a job in an especially pleasant and prompt manner.

9. Be sure to tell the child that chips will only be given for jobs that are done on the first request. If you have to repeat a command to the child, he/she will not receive any chips for doing it.

10. Finally, be sure to go out of your way this week to give chips away for any small appropriate behavior. Remember, you can reward a child even for good behaviors that are not on the list of jobs. Be alert for opportunities to reward the child.

Note: Do not take chips away this week for misbehavior!!! You can do that when your therapist tells you to, but otherwise chips are to be used ONLY as rewards this week, not taken away as punishment.

THE HOME POINT SYSTEM

1. Get a notebook and set it up like a checkbook with five columns, one each for the date, the item, deposits, withdrawals, and the running balance. When your child is rewarded with points, write the job in under "item" and enter the amount as a "deposit." Add it to the child's balance. When your child buys a privilege with his/her points, note the privilege under "item," place this amount in the "withdrawal" column, and deduct this amount from the "balance." The program works just like the chip system except that points are recorded in the book instead of using poker chips.

(*cont.*)

priate time (see below), then return to the child and say, "Are you ready to do as I asked?" If the child did something he/she cannot correct, such as swear or hit, then he/she is simply to promise not to do that again.

8. At this point, the child is to go do what he/she was told to do before going to time out. The parent should then say in a neutral tone of voice, "I like it when you do as I say."

9. Watch for the next appropriate behavior by your child, and then praise the child for it. This ensures that the child always receives as much reward as he/she does punishment in this program and shows him/her that you are not angry at the child but at what the child did.

HOW LONG SHOULD THE CHILD STAY IN TIME OUT?

Your child should stay in time out until three conditions are met:

1. The child must always serve a "minimum sentence" when sent to time out. This should be about 1–2 minutes for each year of his/her age. Use the 1-minute rule for misbehavior that is mild to moderate, and the 2-minute guideline for serious misbehavior.

2. Once the minimum sentence is over, wait until the child is quiet. The first time your child is sent to time out, this may take several minutes to an hour or so. You are not to go to the child until he/she has been quiet for a few moments (about 30 seconds or so), even if it means the child remains in time out for up to 1–2 hours because he/she is arguing, throwing a tantrum, screaming, or crying loudly.

3. Once the child has been quiet for a few moments, the child must agree to do what he/she was told to do. If it was a chore, the child must agree to do it. If it is something the child cannot correct for, such as swearing, lying, and so forth, the child is to promise not to do it again. If the child fails to agree to do what he/she was told (says, "No!"), then tell the child he/she is to sit in the chair until you say he/she can leave. The child is then to serve another minimum sentence, then become quiet, and then agree to do what was asked. The child is not to leave the chair until he/she has agreed to obey the command originally given.

WHAT IF THE CHILD LEAVES THE CHAIR WITHOUT PERMISSION?

Many children will test their parents' authority when time out is first used. They will try to escape from the chair before time is up. Your therapist will discuss with you what actions you should take in punishing your child for leaving the chair. We recommend that the following be done:

1. The first time the child leaves the chair, put him/her back in the chair and say loudly and with a stern appearance, "If you get out of that chair again, I am going to put you in your room!!"

2. When the child leaves the chair again, you are to send the child to his/her bedroom and have the child sit on his/her bed. Be sure that you have removed all of the major play

(cont.)

items from your child's bedroom before using this procedure so that there is little or nothing attractive to play with while the child is in the room.

3. You may leave the door of the child's bedroom open but if the child attempts to leave the room, the door is to be closed and locked, if necessary, to ensure that the time out period is served.

If you disagree with this method, then your therapist will discuss other alternatives you may use instead.

WHAT SHOULD I CONSIDER AS "LEAVING THE CHAIR"?

Generally, a child is considered to have left the chair if both buttocks leave the flat seat of the chair. Thus, the child can swivel about in the chair on his/her buttocks and does not have to face the wall, but if his/her buttocks leave the seat of the chair, then the procedure described above is to be followed. Rocking the chair and tipping it over is also considered leaving the chair. The child should be warned about this.

WHERE SHOULD THE CHAIR BE PLACED?

The chair should be a straight-backed, dinette-style chair. It should be placed in a corner far enough away from the wall that the child cannot kick the wall while in the chair. There should be no play objects nearby and the child should not be able to watch television from the chair. Most parents use a corner of a kitchen, first-floor laundry room, the foyer or entry area of a home, the middle or end of a long hallway, or a corner of a living room (not occupied by others). The location should be such that the parents can observe the child while continuing about their business. Do not use bathrooms, closets, or the child's bedroom. Sometimes, the child can be told to sit on a step at the bottom of a stairway going to a second floor of the home, but a chair is usually preferred.

WHAT TO EXPECT THIS WEEK

If your child follows the pattern typical of most behavior problem children, you can expect that he/she will become quite upset when first sent to time out. As a result, the child may become quite angry and vocal while in time out, or may cry because his/her feelings have been hurt. For many children, this prolonged tantrum or crying results in their having to remain in time out well past their "minimum sentence" because they are not yet quiet. They may therefore spend anywhere from 30 minutes to 1 or 2 hours during the first time out before becoming quiet and agreeing to do what was asked of them. With each use of time out after that, you will find your child becoming quiet much sooner. Eventually, the child will be quiet for most or all of the "minimum sentence" and will agree to do what was asked immediately thereafter. You will also find that your child will begin to obey your first commands, or at least your warnings about time out, such that the frequency of time out eventually decreases. However, this may take several weeks to achieve. Try to remember during this first week of time out that you are not harming your child, but helping to

(cont.)

teach him/her better self-control, respect for parental authority, and the ability to follow rules. Your child may not be happy with this method, but then sometimes children must experience unhappiness if they are to learn certain rules expected to be followed within families and society.

REMINDERS

The child is not to leave the time out chair to use the bathroom or get a drink until his/her time is up and he/she has done what was asked. If children are permitted to do so, they will come to use this demand as a means of escaping from time out on each occasion they are placed in the chair. In addition, if a child is placed in time out during a mealtime, the child is to miss that meal or that portion of mealtime that was spent sitting in the chair. No effort is made to prepare the child a special snack later to compensate for having missed the meal. What makes time out effective is what your child misses while in the chair, and so efforts should not be made to make up for anything the child misses while in time out. Your therapist will discuss with you many ploys children use to try to escape the chair before their time is up. Be sure to ask how to handle each one of them.

If you expect your child will become physically aggressive with you when you try to use time out, ask your therapist how to deal with this situation.

You are to use the time out method for only one or two types of noncompliance during the next week. This prevents your child from being punished excessively at the start of this program. Your therapist will explain these restrictions to you.

If you have any problems with this procedure, call your therapist immediately! Your therapist will provide you with telephone numbers where you can reach him/her this week, should you have problems with this method.

If you want to use the time out method for bedtime behavior problems, please wait 1 week before doing so, as you may find such problems diminish by working on other problems first.

Do not use this procedure out of the home until your therapist tells you to do so.

PARENT HANDOUT FOR STEP 7:
ANTICIPATING PROBLEMS—MANAGING CHILDREN IN PUBLIC PLACES

After your child has been trained to comply with commands at home, it will be easier to teach the child to do so in public places such as stores restaurants, shopping malls, and church. The key to managing children successfully in public places is to establish a plan that you will follow in dealing with your child BEFORE you go into the public place and to make sure that your child is aware of this plan. There are three to four easy rules to follow before you enter any public place:

RULE 1: SET UP THE RULES BEFORE ENTERING THE PLACE

Just before you are about to enter a public place, such as a store, STOP!!! Stand aside and let others enter the place, but don't do so until you have reviewed the important rules of conduct with your child. For instance, for a store the rules for a young child might be: "Stand close, don't touch, and don't beg." For an older child, they might be: "Stay next to me, don't ask for anything, and do as I say." Give your child about three or four rules to follow. These should be rules that are commonly violated by the child in that particular place. After you have told the child the rules, the child is to say them back to you. You and your child are not to enter the place until the child has said these rules. If your child refuses to say them, then warn the child that he/she will be placed in time out in the car. If the child still refuses, then return to your car and place the child in time out there for failing to comply with your request.

RULE 2: SET UP AN INCENTIVE FOR THE CHILD'S COMPLIANCE

While still standing outside the place, tell your child what he/she will earn for adhering to the rules you have just specified and for behaving appropriately in the place. For children who are on a poker chip or point system, these can be used. For children too young for those systems, take along a small bag of snack food (peanuts, raisins, pretzels, corn chips, etc.) to dispense to your child for good behavior throughout the trip. On occasion, you may wish to promise your child a purchase of some sort at the end of the trip, but this should only be done on rare occasions and for exceptionally good behavior during the trip so the child does not come to expect such a purchase as a routine part of any trip away from home. Some parents occasionally promise the child a special privilege at home after the trip. This is fine, but where possible use your chip or point system, as it allows you to reward the child immediately during the trip for good behavior.

RULE 3: SET UP YOUR PUNISHMENT FOR NONCOMPLIANCE

While still outside the place, tell your child what the punishment will be for not following the rules or for misbehavior. In most cases, this will be the loss of points or chips for minor rule violations and the use of time out for moderate to major misbehavior or noncompliance. Do not be afraid to use the time out method in a public place, as it is the most effective method for teaching the child

(cont.)

to obey rules in such places. After you have explained the punishment to the child, then you may enter the public place. Upon doing so, you should begin immediately to do two things: Look around the public place for a convenient time out location if you should need one, and begin attending to and praising your child for following the rules.

If you are using your poker chip or point system, you should give chips or points to your child periodically throughout the trip rather than waiting until the end to provide the reward. In addition, frequent praise and attention should be given to the child for obeying the rules.

RULE 4: GIVE YOUR CHILD AN ACTIVITY TO DO

If possible, think of some activity that your child can do or help with while in this public place so as to occupy his/her time. Part of the reason children misbehave in stores is that they have nothing constructive or helpful to do. This gives them ample time to get into things they shouldn't or find ways to behave foolishly, often only to entertain themselves during the trip. If you are shopping, give your child activities to do to help with the shopping. Any activity you assign your child to do is better than nothing, so even if you have to make up some activity that is not totally constructive, assign something for your child to do.

IN THE PUBLIC PLACE

Once you enter the public place, identify where you will give your child time out, if necessary. Then start to reward him/her with tokens periodically for listening and obeying the rules. If your child starts to misbehave, IMMEDIATELY take away chips/points or place the child in time out. Do not repeat commands or warnings to the child, as the child was already forewarned outside the store as to what would happen if he/she misbehaved. Here are some convenient time out places:

In Department Stores: Take the child to an aisle that is not used much by others and place the child facing a dull side of a display counter or a corner; take the child to the coat section and have him/her face the coat rack; use the gift wrap/credit department area where there is a dull corner; use a dull corner of a restroom; use a changing or dressing room, if nearby; use a maternity section (these are usually not very busy and there are sympathetic moms there).

In Grocery Stores: Have the child face the side of a frozen foods counter; take the child to the furthest corner of the store; find the greeting card display and have the child face the dull side of the counter while you look at cards. It is difficult to find a time out place in most grocery stores, so you may have to use one of the alternatives to time out listed below.

In Church: Take the child to the "crying room" often found in most churches, where mothers take irritable babies during the service; use the foyer or entryway to the church; use a restroom off the lobby of the church.

In a Restaurant: Use the restrooms. Otherwise, use one of the alternatives listed below.

When in Another's Home: Be sure to explain to your hosts that you are using a new child management method and you may need to place your child in a chair or stand the child in a dull corner

(cont.)

somewhere if misbehavior develops. Ask them where one could be used. If this cannot be done in the other's home, then use one of the alternatives listed below.

During a Long Car Trip: Review the rules with the child and set up your incentive before having the child enter the car. Be sure to take along games or activities for the child to do during the trip. If you need to punish the child, pull off the road to a safe stopping area and have the child serve the time out on the floor of the back seat or seated outside the car on a floor mat near the car. Never leave the child in the car unattended and never leave your child unsupervised if he/she is sitting outside the car.

If you use time out in a public place, the minimum sentence needs to be only one-half what it normally is at home, because time out in public places is very effective with children. Also, if the child leaves time out without permission, take away tokens or points as part of his/her token system.

IF YOU CANNOT USE TIME OUT IN THE PUBLIC PLACE

There are always a few places where placing your child in a corner for misbehavior is not possible. Here are some alternatives, but they should be used only where you cannot find a time out area:

1. Take the child outside of the building and have him/her face the wall.

2. Take the child back to your car and have him/her sit on the floor of the back seat. Stay beside the child or in the front seat of the car.

3. Take along a small spiral notepad. Before entering the public place, tell the child that you will write down any episode of misbehavior and the child will then have to go to time out as soon as you get home for any misbehavior. You will find it helpful to take a picture of the child when he/she is in time out at home and keep this with your notepad. Show this picture to the child in front of the public place and explain that this is where he/she can expect to go when you return home if he/she misbehaves.

4. Take along a ballpoint or felt-tip pen. Tell the child in front of the public place that if he/she misbehaves, you will place a hash mark on the back of the child's hand. The child will then serve a minimum sentence in time out at home for each hash mark on the hand.

Important reminder: Whenever you are out with your child, be sure to **act quickly** to deal with misbehavior so that it does not escalate into a loud confrontation with the child or a temper tantrum. Also, be sure to give frequent praise and rewards throughout the trip to reinforce your child's good behavior.

PARENT HANDOUT FOR STEP 8:
USING A DAILY SCHOOL BEHAVIOR REPORT CARD

A daily school behavior report card involves having the teacher send home an evaluation of your child's behavior in school that day, which can be used by you to give or take away rewards available at home. These cards have been shown to be effective in modifying a wide range of problems with children at school. Due to their convenience and cost effectiveness and the fact that they involve both the teacher(s) and parents, they are often one of the first interventions you should try if behavior problems at school are occurring with your child. The teacher reports can consist of either a note or a more formal report card. We recommend the use of a formal behavior report card like those shown at the end of this handout. The card should list the "target" behavior(s) that are to be the focus of the program on the left-hand side of the card. Across the top should be numbered columns that correspond to each class period at school. The teacher gives a number rating reflecting how well the child did for each of these behaviors for each class period. Some examples are provided at the end of this handout.

HOW THE DAILY REPORT CARD WORKS

Using this system, teacher reports are typically sent home on a daily basis. As the child's behavior improves, the daily reports can be reduced to twice weekly (Wednesdays and Fridays), once weekly, or even monthly, and finally phased out altogether. A variety of daily report cards may be developed and tailored for your child. Some of the behaviors targeted for the program may include both social conduct (shares, plays well with peers, follows rules) and academic performance (completes math or reading assignments). Targeting low academic performance (poor production of work) may be especially effective. Examples of behaviors to target include completing all (or a specified portion of) work, staying in the assigned seat, following teacher directions, and playing cooperatively with others. Negative behaviors (e.g., aggression, destruction, calling out) may also be included as target behaviors to be reduced by the program. In addition to targeting class performance, homework may be included. Children sometimes have difficulty remembering to bring homework assignments home. They may also complete their homework but forget to return the completed work to school the next day. Each of these areas may be targeted in a school behavior report card program.

It is recommended that the number of target behaviors you work on be kept to about four or five. Start out by focusing on just a few behaviors you wish to change, to help maximize your child's success in the program. When these behaviors are going well, you can add a few more problem behaviors as targets for change. We recommend including at least one or two positive behaviors that the child is currently doing well with, so that the child will be able to earn some points during the beginning of the program.

Typically, children are monitored throughout the school day. However, to be successful with problem behaviors that occur very frequently, you may want to have the child initially rated for only a

(cont.)

portion of the school day, such as for one or two subjects or classes. As the child's behavior improves, the card can be expanded gradually to include more periods/subjects until the child is being monitored throughout the day. In cases where children attend several different classes taught by different teachers, the program may involve some or all of the teachers, depending on the need for help in each of the classes. When more than one teacher is included in the program, a single report card may include space for all teachers to rate the child. Alternatively, different report cards may be used for each class and organized in a notebook for children to carry between classes. Again, the card shown at the end of this handout can be helpful because it has columns that can be used to rate the child by the same teacher at the end of each subject, or by different teachers.

The success of the program depends on a clear, consistent method for translating the teacher's reports into consequences at home. One advantage of school behavior report cards is that a wide variety of consequences can be used. At a minimum, praise and positive attention should be provided at home whenever a child does well that day at school, as shown on the report card. With many children, however, tangible rewards or token programs are often necessary. For example, a positive note home may translate into television time, a special snack, or a later bedtime. A token system may also be used in which a child earns points for positive behavior ratings and loses points for negative ratings. Both daily rewards (e.g., time with parent, special dessert, television time) and weekly rewards (e.g., movie, dinner at a restaurant, special outing) may be included in the program.

ADVANTAGES OF THE DAILY REPORT CARD

Overall, daily school behavior report cards can be as or even more effective than classroom-based behavior management programs, with effectiveness increased when combined with classroom-based programs. Daily reports seem particularly well suited for children because the children often benefit from the more frequent feedback than is usually provided at school. These programs also give parents more frequent feedback than would normally be provided by the child. As you know, most children, when asked how their school day went, give you a one-word answer, "Fine," which may not be accurate. These report card programs also can remind parents when to reward a child's behavior, and forewarn parents when behavior is becoming a problem at school and will require more intensive work. In addition, the type and quality of rewards available in the home are usually far more extensive than those available in the classroom, a factor that may be critical with children who need more powerful rewards.

Aside from these benefits, daily school report cards generally require much less time and effort from your child's teacher than do classroom-based programs. As a result, teachers who have been unable to start a classroom management program may be far more likely to cooperate with a daily report card that comes from home.

Despite the impressive success of report card programs, the effectiveness of the program depends on the teacher accurately evaluating the child's behavior. It also hinges on the fair and consistent use of consequences at home. In some cases, children may attempt to undercut the system by failing to bring home a report. They may forge a teacher's signature or fail to get a certain teacher's

(cont.)

signature. To discourage these practices, missing notes or signatures should be treated the same way as a "bad" report (i.e., child fails to earn points or is fined by losing privileges or points). The child may even be grounded for the day (no privileges) for not bringing the card home.

SOME EXAMPLES OF DAILY SCHOOL REPORT CARDS

Several types of school behavior report cards that rely on daily school behavior ratings will be discussed here. Two examples are provided at the end of this handout. These are the cards we recommend most parents use if they want to start a school behavior report card quickly. One card is for classroom behavior, the other is for recess behavior. Use whichever card is most appropriate for the problems your child is having at school. Two sets of each card are provided so that you can make photocopies of that page and then cut the page in half to make double the number of cards.

Notice that each card contains five areas of potential behavior problems that children may experience. For the class behavior report card, columns are provided for up to seven different teachers to rate the child in these areas of behavior or for one teacher to rate the child many times across the school day. We have found that the more frequent the ratings, the more effective is the feedback for the children and the more informative the program is to you. The teacher initials the bottom of the column after rating the child's performance during that class period to ensure against forgery. If getting the correct homework assignment home is a problem for some children, the teacher can require the child to copy the homework for that class period on the back of the card before completing the ratings for that period. In this way, the teacher merely checks the back of the card for the child's accuracy in copying the assignment and then completes the ratings on the front of the card. For particularly negative ratings, we also encourage teachers to provide a brief explanation to you as to what resulted in that negative mark. The teachers rate the children using a 5-point system (1 = excellent, 2 = good, 3 = fair, 4 = poor, and 5 = very poor).

The child takes a new card to school each day. These can be kept at school and a new card given out each morning, or you can provide the card as your child leaves for school, whichever is most likely to be done consistently. As soon as the child returns home, you should immediately inspect the card, discuss the positive ratings first with your child, and then proceed to a neutral, business-like (not angry!) discussion with your child about any negative marks and the reason for them. Your child should then be asked to formulate a plan for how to avoid getting a negative mark tomorrow. You are to remind your child of this plan the next morning before your child departs for school. After the child formulates the plan, you should award your child points for each rating on the card and deduct points for each negative mark. For instance, a young elementary school aged child may receive five chips for a 1, three for a 2, and one chip for a 3, while being fined three chips for a 4 and five chips for a 5 on the card. For older children, the points might be 25, 15, 5, –15, and –25, respectively, for marks 1–5 on the card. The chips or points are then added up, the fines are subtracted, and the child may then spend what is left of these chips on the privileges on the home reward menu.

Another daily report card program is provided for dealing with behavior problems and getting along with others during school recess periods or free time periods each day. Again, two cards

(cont.)

are provided on the page so that you can make photocopies of the page and cut the pages in half to double the number of cards. The card is to be completed by the teacher on recess duty during each recess or free time period. It is inspected by the class teacher when the child returns to the classroom, and then should be sent home for use, as above, in a home chip/point system. The classroom teacher should also be instructed to use a "think aloud–think ahead" procedure with the child just prior to the child's going out for recess or free time. In this procedure, the teacher (1) reviews the rules for proper recess behavior with the child and notes that they are written on the card, (2) reminds the child that he/she is being watched by the teacher on recess duty, and (3) directs the child to give the card immediately to the recess monitor so the monitor can evaluate the child's behavior during recess or free time.

As these cards illustrate, virtually any child behavior can be the target for treatment using behavior report cards. If the cards shown here are not suited for your child's behavior problems at school, then design a new card with the assistance of your therapist, using the blank cards provided at the end of this handout. They do not take long to construct and can be very helpful in improving a child's school behavior and performance.

DAILY SCHOOL BEHAVIOR REPORT CARD

Child's name_____ Date_____

Teachers:

Please rate this child's behavior today in the areas listed below. Use a separate column for each subject or class period. Use the following ratings: 1 = excellent, 2 = good, 3 = fair, 4 = poor, and 5 = very poor. Then initial the box at the bottom of your column. Add any comments about the child's behavior today on the back of this card.

	Class periods/subjects						
Behaviors to be rated:	1	2	3	4	5	6	7
Class participation							
Performance of class work							
Follows classroom rules							
Gets along well with other children							
Quality of homework, if any given							
Teacher's initials							

Place comments on back of card

- Cut here after photocopying -

DAILY SCHOOL BEHAVIOR REPORT CARD

Child's name_____ Date_____

Teachers:

Please rate this child's behavior today in the areas listed below. Use a separate column for each subject or class period. Use the following ratings: 1 = excellent, 2 = good, 3 = fair, 4 = poor, and 5 = very poor. Then initial the box at the bottom of your column. Add any comments about the child's behavior today on the back of this card.

	Class periods/subjects						
Behaviors to be rated:	1	2	3	4	5	6	7
Class participation							
Performance of class work							
Follows classroom rules							
Gets along well with other children							
Quality of homework, if any given							
Teacher's initials							

Place comments on back of card

DAILY RECESS AND FREE TIME BEHAVIOR REPORT CARD

Child's name_____ Date_____

Teachers:

Please rate this child's behavior today during recess or other free time periods in the areas listed below. Use a separate column for each recess/free time period. Use the following ratings: 1 = excellent, 2 = good, 3 = fair, 4 = poor, and 5 = very poor. Then initial at the bottom of the column. Add any comments on the back.

Behaviors to be rated:	Recess and free time periods				
	1	2	3	4	5
Keeps hands to self; does not push, shove					
Does not tease others; no taunting/put-downs					
Follows recess/free time rules					
Gets along well with other children					
Does not fight or hit; no kicking or punching					
Teacher's initials					

Place comments on back of card

- Cut here after photocopying -

DAILY RECESS AND FREE TIME BEHAVIOR REPORT CARD

Child's name_____ Date_____

Teachers:

Please rate this child's behavior today during recess or other free time periods in the areas listed below. Use a separate column for each recess/free time period. Use the following ratings: 1 = excellent, 2 = good, 3 = fair, 4 = poor, and 5 = very poor. Then initial at the bottom of the column. Add any comments on the back.

Behaviors to be rated:	Daily recess and free time periods				
	1	2	3	4	5
Keeps hands to self; does not push, shove					
Does not tease others; no taunting/put-downs					
Follows recess or free time rules					
Gets along well with other children					
Does not fight or hit; no kicking or punching					
Teacher's initials					

Place comments on back of card

DAILY SCHOOL BEHAVIOR REPORT CARD

Child's name_____ Date_____

Teachers:

Please rate this child's behavior today in the areas listed below. Use a separate column for each subject or class period. Use the following ratings: 1 = excellent, 2 = good, 3 = fair, 4 = poor, and 5 = very poor. Then initial the box at the bottom of your column. Add any comments about the child's behavior today on the back of this card.

	Class periods/subjects						
Behaviors to be rated:	1	2	3	4	5	6	7
_____							
_____							
_____							
_____							
Teacher's initials							

Place comments on back of card

- Cut here after photocopying -

DAILY SCHOOL BEHAVIOR REPORT CARD

Child's name_____ Date_____

Teachers:

Please rate this child's behavior today in the areas listed below. Use a separate column for each subject or class period. Use the following ratings: 1 = excellent, 2 = good, 3 = fair, 4 = poor, and 5 = very poor. Then initial the box at the bottom of your column. Add any comments about the child's behavior today on the back of this card.

	Class periods/subjects						
Behaviors to be rated:	1	2	3	4	5	6	7
_____							
_____							
_____							
_____							
Teacher's initials							

Place comments on back of card

PARENT HANDOUT FOR STEP 9: MANAGING FUTURE BEHAVIOR PROBLEMS

At this point, you have learned a wide variety of methods for rewarding or punishing your child's behavior. Hopefully, you have found these methods to be effective in improving your child's conduct. However, all children occasionally develop behavior problems, and there is no reason to think that your child will not occasionally develop new problems as he/she grows up. You now have the skills to deal with these problems if you will simply take the time to think about them and set up your own management program. Here are some steps to follow if a new problem develops or an old problem returns:

1. Take out a notebook and begin recording the behavior problem. Try to be specific about what your child is doing wrong. You should record the rule you asked the child to follow that is now being broken, what exactly he/she is doing wrong, and what you are now doing to manage it.

2. Keep this record for a week or so. Then examine it to see what clues it may give you about how to deal with the problem. Many parents find they have returned to some of their old, ineffective habits of dealing with the child and that this has caused the problem. Here are some common mistakes to which parents return:

   a. Repeating your commands too often.
   b. Not giving effective commands (see Step 3).
   c. Not providing attention, praise, or a reward to the child for following the rule correctly. You have stopped your poker chip or points system too early.
   d. Not providing discipline immediately for the rule violation.
   e. Stopping your special playtime with the child.

   Obviously, if you find yourself slipping back into these old habits, correct them. Go back and review your handouts from this program to make sure you are using the methods properly.

3. If you need to, set up a special program for managing the problem:

   a. Explain to your child exactly what you expect her/him to be doing in the problem situation.
   b. Set up a poker chip or point system to reward the child for following the rules.
   c. Use time out immediately each time the problem behavior occurs.
   d. If your notes indicate that the problem seems to be occurring in one particular place or situation, then follow the four steps you were taught to use for public places: (1) anticipate the problem, (2) review the rules just before the problem develops, (3) review the incentives for good behavior, and (4) review the punishment for misbehavior with your child.
   e. Keep recording the behavior problem in your notebook so you can tell when it begins to improve.

4. If these methods fail to work, call your therapist for an appointment and bring along your notes.

References

Abidin, R. R. (1986). *The Parenting Stress Index*. Charlottesville, VA: Pediatric Psychology Press.

Abikoff, H., & Hechtman, L. (1995, June). *Preliminary results of a multi-modal treatment program for ADHD children.* Paper presented at the annual meeting of the International Society for Research in Child and Adolescent Psychopathology, London, England.

Achenbach, T. M. (1991). *Child Behavior Checklist—Cross-Informant Version*. Burlington, VT: Thomas Achenbach.

Achenbach, T. M., & Edelbrock, C. (1983). *Manual for the Child Behavior Checklist and Revised Child Behavior Profile*. Burlington, VT: Thomas Achenbach.

Achenbach, T. M., & Edelbrock, C. (1986). *Manual for the Teacher Report Form and the Child Behavior Profile*. Burlington, VT: Thomas Achenbach.

Achenbach, T. M., & Edelbrock, C. (1987). *Manual for the Child Behavior Checklist Youth Self-Report*. Burlington, VT: Thomas Achenbach.

Achenbach, T. M., McConaughy, S. H., & Howell, C. T. (1987). Child/adolescent behavioral and emotional problems: Implications of cross-informant correlations for situational specificity. *Psychological Bulletin, 101*, 213–232.

Adams, G. L. (1984). *Normative Adaptive Behavior Checklist*. San Antonio, TX: Psychological Corporation.

Adesso, V. J., & Lipson, J. W. (1981). Group training of parents as therapists for their children. *Behavior Therapy, 12*, 625–633.

Altepeter, T. S., & Breen, M. J. (1992). Situational variation in problem behavior at home and school in attention deficit disorder with hyperactivity: A factor analytic study. *Journal of Child Psychology and Psychiatry, 33*, 741–748.

American Psychiatric Association. (1987). *Diagnostic and statistical manual of mental disorders* (3rd ed., rev.). Washington, DC: Author.

American Psychiatric Association. (1994). *Diagnostic and statistical manual of mental disorders* (4th ed.). Washington, DC: Author.

Americans with Disabilities Act of 1990, 42 U.S.C.A. § 12101 *et seq.* (West 1993).

Anastopoulos, A. D., Guevremont, D. C., Shelton, T. L., & DuPaul, G. J. (1992). Parenting stress among families of children with attention deficit hyperactivity disorder. *Journal of Abnormal Child Psychology, 20*, 503–520.

Anastopoulos, A. D., Shelton, T. L., DuPaul, G. J., & Guevremont, D. C. (1993). Parent training for attention-deficit hyperactivity disorder: Its impact on parent functioning. *Journal of Abnormal Child Psychology, 21*, 581–596.

Anderson, J. C., Williams, S., McGee, R., & Silva, P. A. (1987). DSM-III disorders in preadolescent children. *Archives of General Psychiatry, 44,* 69–78.

Applegate, B., Lahey, B. B., Hart, E. L., Waldman, I., Biederman, J., Hynd, G. W., Barkley, R. A., Ollendick, T., Frick, P. J., Greenhill, L., McBurnett, K., Newcorn, J., Kerdyk, L., Garfinkel, B., & Shaffer, D. (1995). *The age of onset for DSM-IV Attention-Deficit/Hyperactivity Disorder: A report of the DSM-IV field trials.* Manuscript submitted for publication.

Asher, S. R., & Coie, J. D. (1990). *Peer rejection in childhood.* New York: Cambridge University Press.

Atkeson, B. M., & Forehand, R. (1978). Parent behavioral training for problem children: An examination of studies using multiple outcome measures. *Journal of Abnormal Child Psychology, 6,* 449–460.

Atkins, M. S., & Pelham, W. E. (1992). School-based assessment of attention-deficit hyperactivity disorder. In S. E. Shaywitz & B. A. Shaywitz (Eds.), *Attention deficit disorder comes of age: Toward the twenty-first century* (pp. 69–88). Austin, TX: Pro-Ed.

Bard, J. (1980). *Rational—emotive therapy in practice.* Champaign, IL: Research Press.

Barkley, R. A. (1981). *Hyperactive children: A handbook for diagnosis and treatment.* New York: Guilford Press.

Barkley, R. A. (1985). The social interactions of hyperactive children: Developmental changes, drug effects, and situational variation. In R. McMahon & R. Peters (Eds.), *Childhood disorders: Behavioral—developmental approaches* (pp. 218–243). New York: Brunner/Mazel.

Barkley, R. A. (1987). *Defiant children: A clinician's manual for parent training.* New York: Guilford Press.

Barkley, R. A. (1988). Child behavior rating scales and checklists. In M. Rutter, A. H. Tuma, & I. S. Lann (Ed.) *Assessment and diagnosis in child psychopathology* (pp. 113–155). New York: Guilford Press.

Barkley, R. A. (1990). *Attention-deficit hyperactivity disorder: A handbook for diagnosis and treatment.* New York: Guilford Press.

Barkley, R. A. (1991). *Multimethod intervention with aggressive ADHD children.* National Institute of Mental Health Grant #45714, Washington, DC.

Barkley, R. A. (1995). *Taking charge of ADHD: The complete, authoritative guide for parents.* New York: Guilford Press.

Barkley, R. A. (1996). Attention-deficit/hyperactivity disorder. In E. J. Mash & R. A. Barkley (Eds.), *Child psychopathology* (pp. 63–112). New York: Guilford Press.

Barkley, R. A. (in press). Behavioral inhibition, sustained attention, and executive functions: Constructing a unifying theory of ADHD. *Psychological Bulletin.*

Barkley, R. A., Anastopoulos, A. D., Guevremont, D. G., & Fletcher, K. F. (1992). Adolescents with attention deficit hyperactivity disorder: Mother—adolescent interactions, family beliefs and conflicts, and maternal psychopathology. *Journal of Abnormal Child Psychology, 20,* 263–288.

Barkley, R. A., & Edelbrock, C. S. (1987). Assessing situational variation in children's behavior problems: The Home and School Situations Questionnaires. In R. Prinz (Ed.), *Advances in behavioral assessment of children and families* (Vol. 3, pp. 157–176). Greenwich, CT: JAI.

Barkley, R. A., Fischer, M., Edelbrock, C. S., & Smallish, L. (1990). The adolescent outcome of hyperactive children diagnosed by research criteria: I. An 8-year prospective follow-up study. *Journal of the American Academy of Child and Adolescent Psychiatry, 29,* 546–557.

Barkley, R. A., Fischer, M., Edelbrock, C. S., & Smallish, L. (1991). The adolescent outcome of hyperactive children diagnosed by research criteria: III. Mother—child interactions, family conflicts, and maternal psychopathology. *Journal of Child Psychology and Psychiatry, 32*, 233–256.

Barkley, R. A., Guevremont, D. G., Anastopoulos, A. D., & Fletcher, K. (1992). A comparison of three family therapy programs for treating family conflicts in adolescents with attention-deficit hyperactivity disorder. *Journal of Consulting and Clinical Psychology, 60*, 450–462.

Barkley, R. A., & Murphy, K. R. (1996). Psychological adjustment and adaptive impairments in young adults with ADHD. *Journal of Attention Disorders, 1*, 41–54.

Bean, A. W., & Roberts, M. W. (1981). The effects of time-out release contingencies on changes in child noncompliance. *Journal of Abnormal Child Psychology, 9*, 95–105.

Beck, A. T., Steer, R. A., & Garbin, M. G. (1988). Psychometric properties of the Beck Depression Inventory: Twenty-five years of evaluation. *Clinical Psychology Review, 8*, 77–100.

Bell, R. Q., & Harper, L. V. (1977). *Child effects on adults.* Hillsdael, NJ: Erlbaum.

Bernal, M. E., Klinnert, M. D., & Schultz, L. A. (1980). Outcome evaluation of behavioral parent training and client-centered parent counseling for children with conduct problems. *Journal of Applied Behavior Analysis, 13*, 677–691.

Biederman, J., Faraone, S. V., Keenan, K., & Tsuang, M. T. (1991). Evidence of a familial association between attention deficit disorder and major affective disorders. *Archives of General Psychiatry, 48*, 633–642.

Biederman, J., Faraone, S. V., Millberger, S., Curtis, S., Chen, L., Marrs, A., Ouellette, C., Moore, P., & Spencer, T. (1996). Predictors of persistence and remission of ADHD into adolescence: Results from a four-year prospective follow-up study. *Journal of the American Academy of Child and Adolescent Psychiatry, 35*, 343–351.

Biederman, J., Keenan, K., & Faraone, S. V. (1990). Parent-based diagnosis of attention deficit disorder predicts a diagnosis based on teacher report. *American Journal of Child and Adolescent Psychiatry, 29*, 698–701.

Blum, N. J., Williams, G. E., Friman, P. C., & Christophersen, E. R. (1995). Disciplining young children: The role of verbal instructions and reasoning. *Pediatrics, 96*, 336–341.

Breen, M. J., & Barkley, R. A. (1988). Child psychopathology and parenting stress in girls and boys having attention deficit disorder with hyperactivity. *Journal of Pediatric Psychology, 13*, 265–280.

Calvert, S. C., & McMahon, R. J. (1987). The treatment acceptability of a behavioral parent training program and its components. *Behavior Therapy, 2*, 165–179.

Campbell, S. B. (1990). *Behavior problems in preschool children.* New York: Guilford Press.

Campbell, S. B., & Ewing, L. J. (1990). Follow-up of hard to manage preschoolers: Adjustment at age 9 and predictors of continuing symptoms. *Journal of Child Psychology and Psychiatry, 31*, 871–889.

Capaldi, D. M. (1992). Co-occurrence of conduct problems and depressive symptoms in early adolescent boys: II. A 2-year follow-up at grade 8. *Development and Psychopathology, 4*, 125–144.

Christensen, A., Johnson, S. M., Phillips, S., & Glasgow, R. E. (1980). Cost effectiveness of behavioral family therapy. *Behavior Therapy, 11*, 208–226.

Christophersen, E. R., Barnard, S. R., & Barnard, J. D. (1981). The family training program manual: The home chip system. In R. A. Barkley, *Hyperactive children: A handbook for diagnosis and treatment* (pp. 437–448). New York: Guilford Press.

Conners, C. K. (1990). *The Conners Rating Scales.* North Tonawanda, NY: Multi-Health Systems.

Crits-Cristoph, P., & Mintz, J. (1991). Implications of therapist effects for the design and analysis of comparative studies of psychotherapies. *Journal of Consulting and Clinical Psychology, 59*, 20–26.

Cunningham, C. E., Bremner, R., & Boyle, M. (1995). Large group community-based parenting programs for families of preschoolers at risk for disruptive behavior disorders: Utilization, cost effectiveness, and outcome. *Journal of Child Psychology and Psychiatry, 36*, 1141–1159.

Dadds, M. R., & McHugh, T. A. (1992). Social support and treatment outcome in behavioral family therapy for child conduct problems. *Journal of Consulting and Clinical Psychology, 60*, 252–259.

Dadds, M. R., Schwartz, S., & Sanders, M. R. (1987). Marital discord and treatment outcome in behavioral treatment of child conduct disorders. *Journal of Consulting and Clinical Psychology, 55*, 396–403.

Danforth, J. S., Barkley, R. A., & Stokes, T. F. (1991). Observations of parent–child interactions with hyperactive children: Research and clinical implications. *Clinical Psychology Review, 11*, 703–727.

Dangel, R. F., & Polster, R. A. (Eds.). (1984). *Parent training: Foundations of research and practice.* New York: Guilford Press.

Day, D. E., & Roberts, M. W. (1982). An analysis of the physical punishment component of a parent training program. *Journal of Abnormal Child Psychology, 11*, 141–152.

Derogatis, L. (1986). *Manual for the Symptom Checklist 90—Revised (SCL-90-R).* Dallas, TX: Psychological Corporation.

Dishion, T. J., & Patterson, G. R. (1992). Age effects in parent training outcome. *Behavior Therapy, 23*, 719–729.

Dodge, K. A., McClaskey, C. L., & Feldman, E. (1985). A situational approach to the assessment of social competence in children. *Journal of Consulting and Clinical Psychology, 53*, 344–353.

Dubey, D. R., O'Leary, S. G., & Kaufman, K. F. (1983). Training parents of hyperactive children in child management: A comparative outcome study. *Journal of Abnormal Child Psychology, 11*, 229–246.

Dumas, J. E. (1984). Interactional correlates of treatment outcome in behavioral parent training. *Journal of Consulting and Clinical Psychology, 52*, 946–954.

Dumas, J. E., Gibson, J. A., & Albin, J. B. (1989). Behavioral correlates of maternal depressive symptomatology in conduct disordered children. *Journal of Consulting and Clinical Psychology, 57*, 516–521.

Dumas, J. E., & Wahler, R. G. (1983). Predictors of treatment outcome in parent training: Mother insularity and socioeconomic disadvantage. *Behavioral Assessment, 5*, 301–313.

Dumas, J. E., & Wahler, R. G. (1985). Indiscriminate mothering as a contextual factor in aggressive–oppositional child behavior: "Damned if you do and damned if you don't." *Journal of Abnormal Child Psychology, 13*, 1–17.

DuPaul, G. R. (1991). Parent and teacher ratings of ADHD symptoms: Psychometric properties in a community-based sample. *Journal of Clinical Child Psychology, 20*, 245–253.

DuPaul, G. J., Anastopoulos, A. D., Power, T. J., Reid, R., Ikeda, M. J., & McGoey, K. E. (1996). *Parent ratings of attention-deficit/hyperactivity disorder symptoms: Factor structure, normative data, and psychometric properties.* Manuscript submitted for publication.

DuPaul, G. J., & Barkley, R. A. (1992). Situational variability of attention problems: Psychometric properties of the Revised Home and School Situations Questionnaires. *Journal of Clinical Child Psychology, 21*, 178–188.

DuPaul, G. J., Barkely, R. A., & McMurray, M. B. (1994). Response of children with ADHD to methylphenidate: Interaction with internalizing symptoms. *Journal of the American Academy of Child and Adolescent Psychiatry, 33*, 894–903.

DuPaul, G. J., Power, T. J., Anastopoulos, A. D., Reid, R., McGoey, K. E., & Ikeda, M. J. (1996).

Teacher ratings of attention-deficit/hyperactivity disorder symptoms: Factor structure, normative data, and psychometric properties. Manuscript submitted for publication.

DuPaul, G. J., Rapport, M. D., & Perriello, L. M. (1991). Teacher ratings of academic skills: The development of the Academic Performance Rating Scale. *School Psychology Review, 20,* 284–300.

DuPaul, G. J., & Stoner, G. (1994). *ADHD in the schools: Assessment and intervention strategies.* New York: Guilford Press.

Dyer, W. (1977). *Your erroneous zones.* New York: Avon.

Ellis, A., & Harper, R. (1975). *A new guide to rational living.* New York: Wilshire.

Evans, S. W., Vallano, M. D., & Pelham, W. (1994). Treatment of parenting behavior with a psychostimulant: A case study of an adult with attention-deficit hyperactivity disorder. *Journal of Child and Adolescent Psychopharmacology, 4,* 63–69.

Eyberg, S. M., & Matarazzo R. G. (1980). Training parents as therapists: A comparison between individual parent–child interaction training and parent group didactic training. *Journal of Clinical Psychology, 36,* 492–499.

Eyberg, S. M., & Robinson, E. A. (1982). Parent–child interaction training: Effects on family functioning. *Journal of Clinical Child Psychology, 11,* 130–137.

Faraone, S. V., Biederman, J., Lehman, B., Keenan, K., Norman, D., Seidman, L. J., Kolodny, R., Kraus, I., Perrin, J., & Chen, W. (1993). Evidence for the independent familial transmission of attention deficit hyperactivity disorder and learning disabilities: Results from a family genetic study. *American Journal of Psychiatry, 150,* 891–895.

Farrington, D. P. (1995). The twelfth Jack Tizard memorial lecture. The development of offending and antisocial behavior from childhood: Key findings from the Cambridge study in delinquent development. *Journal of Child Psychology and Psychiatry, 360,* 929–964.

Fergusson, D. M., Horwood, L. J., & Lynskey, M. T. (1993). Prevalence and comorbidity of DSM-III-R diagnoses in a birth cohort of 15-year-olds. *Journal of the American Academy of Child and Adolescent Psychiatry, 32,* 1127–1133.

Firestone, P., Kelly, M., & Fike, S. (1980). Are fathers necessary in parent training groups? *Journal of Clinical Child Psychology, 44–47.*

Firestone, P., Kelly, M. J., Goodman, J. T., & Davey, J. (1981). Differential effects of parent training and stimulant medication with hyperactives. *Journal of the American Academy of Child Psychiatry, 20,* 135–147.

Firestone, P., & Witt, J. E. (1982). Characteristics of families completing and prematurely discontinuing a behavioral parent training program. *Journal of Pediatric Psychology, 7,* 209–222.

Fischer, M. (1990). Parenting stress and the child with attention deficit hyperactivity disorder. *Journal of Clinical Child Psychology, 19,* 337–346.

Fischer, M., Barkley, R. A., Fletcher, K., & Smallish, L. (1993). The stability of dimensions of behavior in ADHD and normal children over an 8-year period. *Journal of Abnormal Child Psychology, 21,* 315–337.

Fletcher, K., Fischer, M., Barkley, R. A., & Smallish, L. (1996). Sequential analysis of mother–adolescent interactions of ADHD, ADHD/ODD, and normal teenagers during neutral and conflict discussions. *Journal of Abnormal Child Psychology, 24,* 271–297.

Forehand, R. L., & McMahon, R. J. (1981). *Helping the noncompliant child: A clinician's guide to parent training.* New York: Guilford Press.

Forehand, R., & Scarboro, M. E. (1975). An analysis of children's oppositional behavior. *Journal of Abnormal Child Psychology, 3,* 27–31.

Forgatch, M., & Patterson, G. R. (1990). *Parents and adolescents living together.* Eugene, OR: Castalia.

Frankel, F., & Simmons, J. Q., III. (1992). Parent behavioral training: Why and when some parents drop out. *Journal of Clinical Child Psychology, 21,* 322–330.

Frick, P. J., Lahey, B. B., Loeber, R., Stouthamer-Loeber, M., Christ, M. A., & Hanson, K. (1992). Familial risk factors to oppositional defiant disorder and conduct disorder: Parental psychopathology and maternal parenting. *Journal of Consulting and Clinical Psychology, 60,* 49–55.

Frick, P. J., Van Horn, Y., Lahey, B. B., Christ, M. A. G., Loeber, R., Hart, E. A., Tannenbaum, L., & Hanson, K. (1993). Oppositional defiant disorder and conduct disorder: A meta-analytic review of factor analyses and cross-validation in a clinic sample. *Clinical Psychology Review, 13,* 319–340.

Garfield, S. L., & Bergen, A. E. (Eds.). (1986). *Handbook of psychotherapy and behavior change* (3rd ed.). New York: Wiley.

Goldstein, A. P., Keller, H., & Erne, D. (1985). *Changing the abusive parent.* Champaign, IL: Research Press.

Goyette, C. H., Conners, C. K., & Ulrich, R. F. (1978). Normative data for Revised Conners Parent and Teacher Rating Scales. *Journal of Abnormal Child Psychology, 6,* 221–236.

Green, K. D., Forehand, R., & McMahon, R. J. (1979). Parental manipulation of compliance and noncompliance in normal and deviant children. *Behavior Modification, 3,* 245–266.

Greene, R. W., Biederman, J., Faraone, S. V., Ouellette, C. A., Penn, C., & Griffin, S. M. (1996). Toward a new psychometric definition of social disability in children with attention-deficit hyperactivity disorder. *Journal of the American Academy of Child and Adolescent Psychiatry, 35,* 571–578.

Greenhill, L., & Osmon, B. B. (1991). *Ritalin.* New York: Mary Ann Liebert.

Gresham, F., & Elliott, S. (1990). *Social Skills Rating System.* Circle Pines, MN: American Guidance Service.

Haapasalo, J., & Tremblay, R. E. (1994). Physically aggressive boys from ages 6 to 12: Family background, parenting behavior, and prediction of delinquency. *Journal of Consulting and Clinical Psychology, 62,* 1044–1052.

Hefer, R. W., & Kelley, M. L. (1987). Mothers' acceptance of behavioral interventions for children: The influence of parent race and income. *Behavior Therapy, 2,* 153–163.

Hinshaw, S. P. (1987). On the distinction between attentional deficits/hyperactivity and conduct problems/aggression in child psychopathology. *Psychological Bulletin, 101,* 443–463.

Hinshaw, S. P. (1994). *Attention deficits and hyperactivity in children.* Thousand Oaks, CA: Sage.

Hinshaw, S. P., & Anderson, C. A. (1996). Conduct and oppositional defiant disorders. In E. J. Mash & R. A. Barkley (Eds.), *Child psychopathology* (pp. 113–152). New York: Guilford Press.

Hinshaw, S. P., Han, S. S., Erhardt, D., & Huber, A. (1992). Internalizing and externalizing behavior problems in preschool children: Correspondence among parent and teacher ratings and behavior observations. *Journal of Clinical Child Psychology, 21,* 143–150.

Holden, G. W., Lavigne, V. V., & Cameron, A. M. (1990). Probing the continuum of effectiveness in parent training: Characteristics of parents and preschoolers. *Journal of Clinical Child Psychology, 19,* 2–8.

Horn, W. F., Ialongo, N., Greenberg, G., Packard, T., & Smith-Winberry, C. (1990). Additive effects of behavioral parent training and self-control therapy with attention deficit hyperactivity disordered children. *Journal of Clinical Child Psychology, 19,* 98–110.

Horn, W. F., Ialongo, N. S., Pascoe, J. M., Greenberg, G., Packard, T., Lopez, M., Wagner, A., & Puttler, L. (1991). Additive effects of psychostimulants, parent training, and self-control therapy with ADHD children. *Journal of the American Academy of Child and Adolescent Psychiatry, 30,* 233–240.

Horn, W. F., Iolongo, N., Popovich, S., & Peradotto, D. (1987). Behavioral parent training and cognitive-behavioral self-control therapy with ADD-H children: Comparative and combined effects. *Journal of Clinical Child Psychology, 16,* 57–68.

Horton, L. (1984). The father's role in behavioral parent training: A review. *Journal of Clinical Child Psychology, 13,* 274–279.

Humphreys, L., Forehand, R., McMahon, R., & Roberts, M. (1978). Parent behavioral training to modify child noncompliance: Effects on untreated siblings. *Journal of Behavior Therapy and Experimental Psychiatry, 9,* 1–5.

Individuals with Disabilities in Education Act of 1974, 20 U.S.C.A. § 1400 *et seq.*

Jensen, P. S., Watanabe, H. K., Richters, J. E., Cortes, R., Roper, M., & Liu, S. (1995). Prevalence of mental disorder in military children and adolescents: Findings from a two-stage community survey. *Journal of the American Academy of Child and Adolescent Psychiatry, 34,* 1514–1524.

Johnson, S. M., Wahl, G., Martin, S., & Johansson, S. (1973). How deviant is the normal child? A behavioral analysis of the preschool child and his family. In R. D. Rubin, J. P. Brady, & J. D. Henderson (Eds.), *Advances in behavior therapy* (Vol. 4). New York: Academic Press.

Johnston, C. (1992, February). *The influence of behavioral parent training on inattentive overactive and aggressive–defiant behaviors in ADHD children.* Paper presented at the annual meeting of the Society for Research in Child and Adolescent Psychopathology,

Johnston, C. (1996). Parent characteristics and parent–child interactions in families of nonproblem children and ADHD children with higher and lower levels of oppositional–defiant behavior. *Journal of Abnormal Child Psychology, 24,* 85–104.

Kazdin, A. E. (1980). Acceptability of time out from reinforcement procedures for disruptive child behavior. *Behavior Therapy, 11,* 329–344.

Kazdin, A. E. (1991). Effectiveness of psychotherapy with children and adolescents. *Journal of Consulting and Clinical Psychology, 58,* 729–740.

Kazdin, A. E., Esveldt-Dawson, K., French, N. H., & Unis, A. S. (1987). Effects of parent management training and problem-solving skills training combined in the treatment of antisocial child behavior. *Journal of the American Academy of Child and Adolescent Psychiatry, 26,* 416–424.

Kazdin, A. E., Siegel, T. C., & Bass, D. (1992). Cognitive problem-solving skills training and parent management training in the treatment of antisocial behavior in children. *Journal of Consulting and Clinical Psychology, 60,* 733–747.

Keenan, K., & Shaw, D. S. (1994). The development of aggression in toddlers: A study of low-income families. *Journal of Abnormal Child Psychology, 22,* 53–77.

Kelley, M. L., Embry, L. H., & Baer, D. M. (1979). Skills for child management and family support. *Behavior Modification, 3,* 373–396.

Knapp, P. A., & Deluty, R. H. (1989). Relative effectiveness of two behavioral parent training programs. *Journal of Clinical Child Psychology, 18,* 314–322.

Lachar, D. (1982). *Personality Inventory for Children (PIC): Revised format manual supplement.* Los Angeles: Western Psychological Services.

Lahey, B. B., Applegate, B., Barkley, R. A., Garfinkel, B., McBurnett, K., Lerdyk, L., Greenhill, L., Hynd, G. W., Frick, P. J., Newcorn, J., Biederman, J., Ollendick, T., Hart, E. L., Perez, D., Waldman, I., & Shaffer, D. (1994). DSM-IV field trials for Oppositional Defiant Disorder and Conduct Disorder in children and adolescents. *American Journal of Psychiatry, 151,* 1163–1171.

Lahey, B. B., Applegate, B., McBurnett, K., Biederman, J., Greenhill, L., Hynd, G. W., Barkley, R. A., Newcorn, J., Jensen, P., Richters, J., Garfinkel, B., Kerdyk, L., Frick, P. J., Ollendick, T., Perez, D., Hart, E., Waldman, I., & Shaffer, D. (1994). DSM-IV field trials for Attention Deficit Hyperactivity Disorder in children and adolescents. *American Journal of Psychiatry*, *151*, 1673–1685.

Lahey, B. B., & Loeber, R. (1994). Framework for a developmental model of oppositional defiant disorder and conduct disorder. In D. K. Routh (Ed.), *Disruptive behavior disorders in childhood* (pp. 139–180). New York: Plenum Press.

Lahey, B. B., Loeber, R., Quay, H. C., Frick, P. J., & Grimm, J. (1992). Oppositional defiant and conduct disorders: Issues to be resolved for DSM-IV. *Journal of the American Academy of Child and Adolescent Psychiatry*, *31*, 539–546.

Lahey, B. B., Piacentini, J. C., McBurnett, K., Stone, P., Hartdagen, S., & Hynd, G. W. (1988). Psychopathology in the parents of children with conduct disorder and hyperactivity. *Journal of the American Academy of Child and Adolescent Psychiatry*, *27*, 163–170.

Larzelere, R. E. (1996). *A review of the outcomes of parental use of nonabusive or customary physical punishment*. Paper presented at the meeting of the American Academy of Pediatrics, San Francisco.

Latham, P., & Latham, R. (1992). *ADD and the law*. Washington, DC: JKL Communications.

Lewinsohn, P. M., Hops, H., Roberts, R. E., Seeley, J. R., & Andrews, J. A. (1993). Adolescent psychopathology: I. Prevalence and incidence of depression and other DSM-III-R disorders in high school students. *Journal of Abnormal Psychology*, *102*, 133–144.

Lilienfeld, S. O., & Marino, L. (1995). Mental disorder as a Roschian concept: A critique of Wakefield's "harmful dysfunction" analysis. *Journal of Abnormal Psychology*, *104*, 411–420.

Little, L. M., & Kelley, M. L. (1989). The efficacy of response cost procedures for reducing children's noncompliance to parental instructions. *Behavior Therapy*, *20*, 515–534.

Locke, H. J., & Wallace, K. M. (1959). Short marital adjustment and prediction tests: Their reliability and validity. *Journal of Marriage and Family Living*, *21*, 251–255.

Loeber, R. (1988). Natural histories of conduct problems, delinquency, and associated substance use. In B. B. Lahey & A. E. Kazdin (Eds.), *Advances in clinical child psychology* (Vol. 11, pp. 73–124). New York: Plenum Press.

Loeber, R. (1990). Development and risk factors of juvenile antisocial behavior and delinquency. *Clinical Psychology Review*, *10*, 1–41.

Loeber, R., Green, S. M., Lahey, B. B., Christ, M. A. G., & Frick, P. J. (1992). Developmental sequences in the age of onset of disruptive child behaviors. *Journal of Child and Family Studies*, *1*, 21–41.

Loeber, R., Green, S., Lahey, B. B., & Stouthamer-Loeber, M. (1991). Differences and similarities between children, mothers, and teachers as informants on disruptive behavior disorders. *Journal of Abnormal Child Psychology*, *19*, 75–95.

Loeber, R., Wung, P., Keenan, K., Giroux, B., Stouthamer-Loeber, M., Van Kammen, W. B., & Maughan, B. (1993). Developmental pathways in disruptive child behavior. *Development and Psychopathology*, *5*, 101–131.

Lynskey, M. T., & Fergusson, D. M. (1994). Childhood conduct problems, attention deficit behaviors, and adolescent alcohol, tobacco, and illicit drug use. *Journal of Abnormal Child Psychology*, *23*, 281–302.

Mann, B. J., Borduin, C. M., Henggeler, S. W., & Blaske, D. M. (1990). An investigation of systemic conceptualizations of parent–child coalitions and symptom change. *Journal of Consulting and Clinical Psychology*, *3*, 336–344.

Mann, B. J., & MacKenzie, E. P. (1996). Pathways among marital functioning, parental behaviors, and child behavior problems in school-age boys. *Journal of Clinical Child Psychology*, *25*, 183–191.

Martin, B. (1977). Brief family intervention: Effectiveness and the importance of including the father. *Journal of Consulting and Clinical Psychology*, *45*, 1002–1010.

Mash, E. J., & Barkley, R. A. (Eds.). (1989). *Treatment of childhood disorders*. New York: Guilford Press.

Mash, E. J., & Barkley, R. A. (Eds.). (1996). *Child psychopathology*. New York: Guilford Press.

Mash, E. J., & Barkley, R. A. (Eds.). (in press). *Treatment of childhood disorders* (2nd ed.). New York: Guilford Press.

Mash, E. J., & Dozois, D. J. A. (1996). Child psychopathology: A developmental systems perspective. In E. J. Mash & R. A. Barkley (Eds.), *Child psychopathology* (pp. 3–62). New York: Guilford Press.

Mash, E. J., Hamerlynck, L. A., & Handy, L. C. (1976). *Behavior modification and families*. New York: Brunner/Mazel.

Mash, E. J., Handy, L. C., & Hamerlynck, L. (1976). *Behavior modification approaches to parenting*. New York: Brunner/Mazel.

Mash, E. J., & Johnston, C. (1982). A comparison of mother–child interactions of younger and older hyperactive and normal children. *Child Development, 53*, 1371–1381.

Mash, E. J., & Johnston, C. (1990). Determinants of parenting stress: Illustrations from families of hyperactive children and families of physically abused children. *Journal of Clinical Child Psychology, 19*, 313–328.

Mash, E. J., & Terdal, L. G. (Eds.). (1997). *Assessment of childhood disorders*. New York: Guilford Press.

Matson, J. L. (1993). *Handbook of hyperactivity in children*. Boston: Allyn & Bacon.

Matson, J. L., Rotatori, A. F., & Helsel, W. J. (1983). Development of a rating scale to measure social skills in children: The Matson Evaluation of Social Skills with Youngsters (MESSY). *Behaviour Research and Therapy, 21*, 335–340.

McGee, R., Feehan, M., Williams, S., Partridge, F., Silva, P. A., & Kelly, J. (1990). DSM-III disorders in a large sample of adolescents. *Journal of the American Academy of Child and Adolescent Psychiatry, 29*, 611–619.

McMahon, R. J., & Forehand, R. (1984). Parent training for the noncompliant child. In R. F. Dangel & R. A. Polster (Eds.), *Parent training: Foundations of research and practice* (pp. 298–328). New York: Guilford Press.

McMahon, R. J., Tiedemann, G. L., Forehand, R., & Griest, D. L. (1984). Parental satisfaction with parent training to modify child noncompliance. *Behavior Therapy, 15*, 295–303.

Moffitt, T. E. (1990). Juvenile delinquency and attention deficit disorder: Boys' developmental trajectories from age 3 to age 15. *Child Development , 61*, 893–910.

Murphy, K. R., & Barkley, R. A. (1996a). ADHD adults: Comorbidities and adaptive impairments. *Comprehensive Psychiatry, 37*, 393–401.

Murphy, K. R., & Barkley, R. A. (1996b). Parents of children with attention-deficit/hyperactivity disorder: Psychological and attentional impairment. *American Journal of Orthopsychiatry, 66*, 93–102.

Murphy, K. R., & Barkley, R. A. (1996c). Prevalence of DSM-IV ADHD symptoms in an adult community sample of licensed drivers. *Journal of Attention Disorders, 1*, 147–161.

Newcomb, A. F., Bukowski, W. M., & Pattee, L. (1993). Children's peer relations: A meta-analytic review of popular, rejected, neglected, controversial, and average sociometric status. *Psychological Bulletin, 113,* 99–128.

Olson, S. L. (1992). Development of conduct problems and peer rejection in preschool children: A social systems analysis. *Journal of Abnormal Child Psychology, 20,* 327–350.

Olweus, D. (1979). Stability of aggressive reaction patterns in males: A review. *Psychological Bulletin, 86,* 852–875.

Olweus, D. (1980). Familial and temperamental determinants of aggressive behavior in adolescent boys: A causal analysis. *Developmental Psychology, 16,* 644–660.

Palfrey, J. S., Levine, M. D., Walker, D. K., & Sullivan, M. (1985). The emergence of attention deficits in early childhood: A prospective study. *Developmental and Behavioral Pediatrics, 6,* 339–348.

Paternite, C., & Loney, J. (1980). Childhood hyperkinesis: Relationships between symptomatology and home environment. In C. K. Whalen & B. Henker (Eds.), *Hyperactive children: The social ecology of identification and treatment* (pp. 105–141). New York: Academic Press.

Patterson, G. R. (1976). The aggressive child: Victim and architect of a coercive system. In E. J. Mash, L. A. Hamerlynck, & L. C. Handy (Eds.), *Behavior modification and families* (pp. 267–316). New York: Bruner/Mazel.

Patterson, G. R. (1982). *Coercive family process.* Eugene, OR: Castalia.

Patterson, G. R., & Chamberlain, P. (1994). A functional analysis of resistance during parent-training therapy. *Clinical Psychology: Science and Practice, 1,* 53–70.

Patterson, G. R., Chamberlain, P., & Reid, J. B. (1982). A comparative evaluation of a parent-training program. *Behavior Therapy, 13,* 638–650.

Patterson, G. R., Dishion, T. J., & Chamberlain, P. (1993). Outcomes and methodological issues relating to treatment of antisocial children. In T. R. Giles (Ed.), *Handbook of effective psychotherapy.* New York: Plenum Press.

Patterson, G. R., & Fleischman, M. J. (1979). Maintenance of treatment effects: Some considerations concerning family systems and follow-up data. *Behavior Therapy, 10,* 168–185.

Patterson, G. R., & Forgatch, M. S. (1985). Therapist behavior as a determinant for client noncompliance: A paradox for the behavior modifier. *Journal of Consulting and Clinical Psychology, 53,* 846–851.

Patterson, G. R., Reid, J. B., & Dishion, T. J. (1992). *Antisocial boys.* Eugene, OR: Castalia.

Patterson, G. R., Reid, J. B., Jones, R. R., & Conger, R. E. (1975). *A social learning approach to family intervention* (Vol. 1). Eugene, OR: Castalia.

Pearson, J. L., Ialongo, N. S., Hunter, A. G., & Kellam, S. G. (1993). Family structure and aggressive behavior in a population of urban elementary school children. *Journal of the American Academy of Child and Adolescent Psychiatry, 33,* 540–548.

Pelham, W. E., Jr., Gnagy, E. M., Greenslade, K. E., & Milich, R. (1992). Teacher ratings of DSM-III symptoms for the disruptive behavior disorders. *Journal of the American Academy of Child and Adolescent Psychiatry, 31,* 210–218.

Pelham, W. E., Jr., & Lang, A. R. (1993). Parental alcohol consumption and deviant child behavior: Laboratory studies of reciprocal effects. *Clinical Psychology Review, 13,* 763–784.

Pfiffner, L. J., Jouriles, E. N., Brown, M. M., Etscheidt, M. A., & Kelly, J. A. (1988, November). *Enhancing the effects of parent training for single-parent families.* Paper presented at the 22nd annual meeting of the Association for Advancement of Behavior Therapy, New York.

Pisterman, S., McGrath, P., Firestone, P., Goodman, J. T., Webster, I., & Mallory, R. (1989). Outcome of parent-mediated treatment of preschoolers with attention deficit disorder with hyperactivity. *Journal of Consulting and Clinical Psychology, 57,* 628–635.

Pollard, S., Ward, E., & Barkley, R. (1983). The effects of parent training and Ritalin on the parent–child interactions of hyperactive boys. *Child and Family Behavior Therapy, 5*, 51–69.

Prinz, R. J., & Miller, G. E. (1994). Family-based treatment for childhood antisocial behavior: Experimental influences on dropout and engagement. *Journal of Consulting and Clinical Psychology, 62*, 645–650.

Prior, M. (1992). Childhood temperament. *Journal of Child Psychology and Psychiatry, 33,* 249–279.

Quici, F. L., Wheeler, S. R., & Bolle, J. (1996, March). *Does training parents of defiant children really work? Seven years of data.* Paper presented at the annual meeting of the National Association of School Psychologists, Atlanta, GA.

Rapport, M. D., & Kelly, K. L. (1993). Psychostimulant effects on learning and cognitive function in children with attention deficit hyperactivity disorder: Findings and implications. In J. L. Matson (Ed.), *Hyperactivity in children: A handbook* (pp. 97–136). New York: Pergamon Press.

Rehabilitation Act of 1973, 29 U.S.C.A. § 701 *et seq.*

Reynolds, C., & Kamphaus, R. (1994). *Behavioral Assessment System for Children.* Circle Pines, MN: American Guidance Service.

Richters, J. E., & Cichetti, D. (1993). Mark Twain meets DSM-III-R: Conduct disorder, development, and the concept of harmful dysfunction. *Development and Psychopathology, 5*, 5–29.

Roberts, M. W. (1982). Resistance to timeout: Some normative data. *Behavioral Assessment, 4*, 237–246.

Roberts, M. W. (1985). Praising child compliance: Reinforcement or ritual? *Journal of Abnormal Child Psychology, 13*, 611–629.

Roberts, M. W., Hatzenbuehler, L. C., & Bean, A. W. (1981). The effects of differential attention and time out on child noncompliance. *Behavior Therapy, 12*, 93–99.

Roberts, M. W., McMahon, R. J., Forehand, R., & Humphreys, L. (1978). The effect of parental instruction-giving on child compliance. *Behavior Therapy, 9*, 793–798.

Robin, A. L. (1979). Problem-solving communication training: A behavioral approach to the treatment of parent–adolescent conflict. *American Journal of Family Therapy, 7*, 69–82.

Robin, A. L. (1981). A controlled evaluation of problem-solving communication training with parent–adolescent conflict. *Behavior Therapy, 12*, 593–609.

Robin, A. L. (1984). Parent–adolescent conflict: A developmental problem of families. In R. McMahon & R. Peters (Eds.), *Childhood disorders: Developmental–behavioral approaches* (pp. 244–266). New York: Brunner/Mazel.

Robin, A. R., & Foster, S. L. (1989). *Negotiating parent–adolescent conflict: A behavioral–family systems approach.* New York: Guilford Press.

Rogers, T. R., Forehand, R., Griest, D. L., Wells, K. C., & McMahon, R. J. (1981). Socioeconomic status: Effects of parent and child behaviors and treatment outcome of parent training. *Journal of Clinical Child Psychology, 10*, 98–101.

Roizen, N. J., Blondis, T. A., Irwin, M., & Stein, M. (1994). Adaptive functioning in children with attention-deficit hyperactivity disorder. *Archives of Pediatric and Adolescent Medicine, 148*, 1137–1142.

Russo, D. C., Cataldo, M. F., & Cushing, P. J. (1981). Compliance training and behavioral covariation in the treatment of multiple behavior problems. *Journal of Applied Behavior Analysis, 14,* 209–222.

Salzinger, S., Kaplan, S., & Artemyeff, C. (1983). Mothers' personal social networks and child maltreatment. *Journal of Abnormal Psychology, 92*, 68–76.

Sanders, M. R. (1996). New directions in behavioral family intervention with children. In T. H. Ollendick & R. J. Prinz (Eds.), *Advances in clinical child psychology* (Vol. 18, pp. 283–330). New York: Plenum Press.

Sanders, M. R., & Christensen, A. P. (1984). A comparison of the effects of child management and planned activities training in five parenting environments. *Journal of Abnormal Child Psychology, 13*, 101–117.

Sanders, M. R., & Dadds, M. R. (1982). The effects of planned activities and child management procedures in parent training: An analysis of setting generality. *Behavior Therapy, 13*, 452–461.

Sanders, M. R., & Glynn, T. (1981). Training parents in behavioral self-management: An analysis of generalization and maintenance. *Journal of Applied Behavior Analysis, 14*, 223–237.

Schachar, R., & Wachsmuth, R. (1990). Oppositional Disorder in children: A validation study comparing Conduct Disorder, Oppositional Disorder and normal control children. *Journal of Child Psychology and Psychiatry, 31*, 1089–1102.

Schaefer, C. E., & Briesmeister, J. M. (1989). *Handbook of parent training*. New York: Wiley.

Shaw, D. S., & Vondra, J. I. (1995). Infant attachment security and maternal predictors of early behavior problems: A longitudinal study of low-income families. *Journal of Abnormal Child Psychology, 23*, 335–357.

Shekim, W., Asarnow, R. F., Hess, E., Zaucha, K., & Wheeler, N. (1990). An evaluation of attention deficit disorder—residual type. *Comprehensive Psychiatry, 31*, 416–425.

Shriver, M. D., & Allen, K. D. (1996). The time-out grid: A guide to effective discipline. *School Psychology Quarterly, 11*, 67–75.

Sleator, E. K., & Ullmann, R. K. (1981). Can the physician diagnose hyperactivity in the office? *Pediatrics, 67*, 13–17.

Snyder, J., & Brown, K. (1983). Oppositional behavior and noncompliance in preschool children: Environmental correlates and skills deficits. *Behavioral Assessment, 5*, 333–348.

Snyder J., & Patterson, G. R. (1995). Individual differences in social aggression: A test of the reinforcement model of socialization in the natural environment. *Behavior Therapy, 26*, 371–391.

Socolar, R. S., & Stein, R. E. K. (1995). Spanking infants and toddlers: Maternal belief and practice. *Pediatrics, 95*, 105–111.

Spaccarelli, S., Cotler, S., & Penman, D. (1992). Problem-solving skills training as a supplement to behavioral parent training. *Cognitive Therapy and Research, 16*, 1–18.

Sparrow, S. S., Baila, D. A., & Cicchetti, D. V. (1984). *Vineland Adaptive Behavior Scales*. Circle Pines, MN: American Guidance Service.

Speltz, M. L., DeKlyen, M., Greenberg, M. T., & Dryden, M. (1995). Clinic referral for oppositional defiant disorder: Relative significance of attachment and behavioral variables. *Journal of Abnormal Child Psychology, 23*, 487–507.

Spitzer, A., Webster-Stratton, C., & Hollinsworth, T. (1991). Coping with conduct-problem children: Parents gaining knowledge and control. *Journal of Clinical Child Psychology, 20*, 413–427.

Stormont-Spurgin, M., & Zentall, S. S. (1995). Contributing factors in the manifestation of aggression in preschoolers with hyperactivity. *Journal of Child Psychology and Psychiatry, 3*, 491–509.

Strain, P. S., Steele, P., Ellis, T., & Timm, M. A. (1982). Long-term effects of oppositional child treatment with mothers as therapists and therapist trainers. *Journal of Applied Behavior Analysis, 15*, 163–169.

Strain, P. S., Young, C. C., & Horowitz, J. (1981). Generalized behavior change during opposi-tional child training: An examination of child and family demographic variables. *Behavior Modification, 5*, 15–26.

Strassberg, Z., Dodge, K. A., Petit, G. S., & Bates, J. E. (1994). Spanking in the home and children's subsequent aggression toward kindergarten peers. *Development and Psychopathol-ogy, 6*, 445–461.

Strayhorn, J. M., & Weidman, C. S. (1989). Reduction of attention deficit and internalizing symptoms in preschoolers through parent–child interaction training. *Journal of the Ameri-can Academy of Child and Adolescent Psychiatry, 28*, 888–896.

Strayhorn, J. M., & Weidman, C. S. (1991). Follow-up one year after parent–child interaction training: Effects on behavior of preschool children. *Journal of the American Academy of Child and Adolescent Psychiatry, 30*, 138–143.

Swanson, J. M., McBurnett, K., Christian, D. L., & Wigal, T. (1995). Stimulant medications and the treatment of children with ADHD. In T. H. Ollendick & R. J. Prinz (Ed.), *Ad-vances in clinical child psychology* (Vol. 17, pp. 265–321). New York: Plenum Press.

Tolan, P. H. (1987). Implications of age of onset for delinquency risk. *Journal of Abnormal Child Psychology, 15*, 47–65.

Tremblay, R. E., Masse, B., Perron, D., Leblanc, M., Schwartzman, A. E., & Ledingham, J. E. (1992). Early disruptive behavior, poor school achievement, delinquent behavior, and de-linquent personality: Longitudinal analyses. *Journal of Consulting and Clinical Psychology, 60*, 65–72.

Tremblay, R. E., Pihl, R. O., Vitaro, F., & Dobkin, P. L. (1994). Predicting early onset of male antisocial behavior from preschool behavior. *Archives of General Psychiatry, 51*, 732–738.

Tschann, J. M., Kaiser, P., Chesney, M. A., Alkon, A., & Boyce, W. T. (1996). Resilience and vulnerability among preschool children: Family functioning, temperament, and behavior problems. *Journal of the American Academy of Child and Adolescent Psychiatry, 35*, 184–191.

Vaden-Kiernan, N., Ialongo, N. S., Pearson, J., & Kellam, S. (1995). Household family struc-ture and children's aggressive behavior: A longitudinal study of urban elementary school children. *Journal of Abnormal Child Psychology, 23*, 553–568.

Vuchinich, S., Bank, L., & Patterson, G. R. (1992). Parenting, peers, and the stability of antiso-cial behavior in preadolescent boys. *Developmental Psychology, 28*, 510–521.

Wahler, R. (1975). Some structural aspects of deviant child behavior. *Journal of Applied Behavior Analysis, 8*, 27–42.

Wahler, R. G. (1980). The insular mother: Her problems in parent–child treatment. *Journal of Applied Behavior Analysis, 13*, 207–219.

Wahler, R. G., & Afton, A. D. (1980). Attentional processes in insular and noninsular mothers: Some differences in their summary reports about child problem behaviors. *Child Behavior Therapy, 2*, 25–41.

Wahler, R. G., Cartor, P. G., Fleischman, J., & Lambert, W. (1993). The impact of synthesis teaching and parent training with mothers of conduct-disordered children. *Journal of Ab-normal Child Psychology, 21*, 425–440.

Wahler, R. G., & Fox, J. J. (1980). Solitary toy play and time out: A family treatment package for children with aggressive and oppositional behavior. *Journal of Applied Behavior Analysis, 13*, 23–39.

Wahler, R. G., & Graves, M. G. (1983). Setting events in social networks: Ally or enemy in child behavior therapy? *Behavior Therapy, 14*, 19–36.

Wakefield, J. C. (1992). Disorder as harmful dysfunction: A conceptual critique of DSM-III-R's definition of mental disorder. *Psychological Review*, 99, 232–247.

Webster-Stratton, C. (1982). The long-term effects of a videotape modeling parent-training program: Comparison of immediate and 1-year follow-up results. *Behavior Therapy*, 13, 702–714.

Webster-Stratton, C. (1984). Randomized trial of two parent-training programs for families with conduct disordered children. *Journal of Consulting and Clinical Psychology*, 52, 666–678.

Webster-Stratton, C. (1991). Stress: A potential disruptor of parent perceptions and family interactions. *Journal of Clinical Child Psychology*, 19, 302–312.

Webster-Stratton, C., & Hammond, M. (1990). Predictors of treatment outcome in parent training for families with conduct problem children. *Behavior Therapy*, 21, 319–337.

Webster-Stratton, C., Hollinsworth, T., & Kolpacoff, M. (1989). The long-term effectiveness and clinical significance of three cost-effective training programs for families with conduct-problem children. *Journal of Consulting and Clinical Psychology*, 57, 550–553.

Webster-Stratton, C., Kolpacoff, M., & Hollinsworth, T. (1995). Self-administered videotape therapy for families with conduct-problem children: Comparison with two cost-effective treatments and a control group. *Journal of Consulting and Clinical Psychology*, 56, 558–566.

Webster-Stratton, C., & Spitzer, A. (1996). Parenting a young child with conduct problems. In T. H. Ollendick & R. J. Prinz (Eds.), *Advances in clinical child psychology* (Vol. 18, pp. 1–62). New York: Plenum Press.

Weiss, G. (1992, October). *Child and adolescent psychiatry clinics of North America: Vol. 1. Attention-Deficit Hyperactivity Disorder*. Philadelphia: Saunders.

Weiss, G., & Hechtman, L. T. (1993). *Hyperactive children grown up* (2nd ed.): *ADHD in children, adolescents, and adults*. New York: Guilford Press.

Wells, K. C., & Forehand, R. (1985). Conduct and Oppositional Disorders. In P. H. Bornstein & A. E. Kazdin (Eds.), *Handbook of clinical behavior therapy with children* (pp. 219–265). Champaign, IL: Dorsey Press.

Wells, K. C., Forehand, R., & Griest, D. L. (1980). Generality of treatment effects from treated to untreated behaviors resulting from a parent training program. *Journal of Clinical Child Psychology*, 9, 217–219.

Wenning, K., Nathan, P., & King, S. (1993). Mood disorders in children with oppositional defiant disorder: A pilot study. *American Journal of Orthopsychiatry*, 63, 295–299.

Werry, J., & Aman, M. (1993). *Practitioner's guide to psychoactive drugs for children and adolescents*. New York: Plenum Press.

Werry, J., & Aman, M. (in press). *Practitioner's guide to psychoactive drugs for children and adolescents* (2nd ed.). New York: Plenum Press.

Williams, C. A., & Forehand, R. (1984). An examination of predictor variables for child compliance and noncompliance. *Journal of Abnormal Child Psychology*, 12, 491–504.

Worland, J., Carney, R., Milich, R., & Grame, C. (1980). Does in-home training add to the effectiveness of operant group parent training? *Child Behavior Therapy*, 2, 11–24.

Wozniak, J., & Biederman, J. (1995). Prepubertal mania exists (and co-exists with ADHD). *ADHD Report*, 2(3), 5–6.

Zoccolillo, M. (1993). Gender and the development of conduct disorder. *Development and Psychopathology*, 5, 65–78.

Abusive families, 3, 37, 48, 68
Academic Performance Rating Scale, 60
Accountability for behavior, 69–70
Activity level of child, 94
Adaptive behavior, 20, 61
Age
  of child, 2–3, 7
    and interview techniques, 54–55
    and outcome of program, 5
    and prevalence of defiance, 26
    in psychiatric disorders, 50, 51, 52
    in time out procedure, 136
    in token system, 122–123, 124
  of parents, 8, 64
Aggressive behavior, 27, 45, 141
Anticipation of problems, 4, 83, 86, 87
  in future, 159–161, 247
  in public, 83, 86, 147–154, 237–239
  in transition periods, 86, 153–154
Antisocial behavior, 19, 41, 42
Anxiety disorders, 45, 199–202
Assessment procedures, 11–12, 44–72
  on adaptive behavior, 61
  behavior rating scales in. *See* Behavior rating
      scales
  cost of, 46, 56
  family screening in, 70–72
  forms used in, 165–214
  interviews in. *See* Interviews
  legal and ethical issues in, 48, 68–70
  objectives of, 44–45
  on peer relationships, 62
  permission requests in, 181, 185
  in posttreatment follow-up, 163
  preparation for, 47, 179–187
  prior to first appointment, 46–47
    forms used in, 167, 169–173
  self-reports in. *See* Self-reports
  treatment implications of, 20–22, 67–68,
      70–72
Attachment relationships, 34
Attention deficit/hyperactivity disorder, 2, 4, 5
  adaptive behavior in, 61
  behavior rating scales in, 58, 59, 60–61
  child interview in, 55
  diagnosis of, 12, 44, 45, 195–197
    criteria in, 23, 25, 51–52
  drug therapy in, 163–164
  duration of symptoms in, 51
  effectiveness of program in, 8
  frequency of referrals for, 27
  intervention criteria in, 20
  legal and ethical issues in, 68, 69
  and oppositional behavior, 9, 40
  in parent, 9–10, 12, 63–64
  parent interview in, 48, 49, 51–53, 195–
      197

peer relationships in, 62
teacher reports on, 52, 56, 57
Attention of parent, 4, 6, 85, 102–119
  to appropriate behavior, 35, 36, 105
  to compliant behavior, 111–119
    handout on, 113, 116–117, 226
    in public places, 151
    in time out procedure, 137
  to disruptive behavior, 116
  inadvertent reinforcement in, 35
  maintenance of treatment gains in, 6
  to play behavior. *See* Play behavior, attention
      of parent to
  supervisor exercise on, 103–104
  in token systems, 124, 128–129
Attention span of child, 94
Avoidance behavior, 30, 97

Behavior rating scales, 57–61
  on adaptive behavior, 61
  adult self-report forms on, 213–214
  for children, 60–61
  for parents and teachers, 57–60
  on peer relationships, 62
  in posttreatment follow-up, 163
  for reevaluation, 92–93, 121, 148
Behavioral Assessment System for Children,
    46, 47, 58, 62
Bipolar disorders, 2, 45, 205–207
Booster sessions, 87, 162–164
Breakage fees, 75–76, 78

Causes of defiant behavior, 39–42, 85, 91–101
  child characteristics in, 39–40, 93–96
    parent handout on, 94–96, 219
  consequences of misbehavior in, 39, 97–98
  contextual factors in, 41–42
  family stress events in, 41, 98–99
  interactions among, 41–42, 99
  model on, 39, 93–99
  parent characteristics in, 39, 40–41, 96–97
  parent–child relationship in, 39
  understanding of parents on, 93
Child Attention Problems Scale, 59
Child Behavior Checklist, 46, 47, 58, 59
  on adaptive behavior, 61
  on peer relationships, 62
  self-report version, 60, 61
Clinic
  behavior of child in, 55–56, 185
  training program in, 74, 79–80
Cognitive characteristics
  of child, 39–40
  of parent, 40–41
Command–compliance interactions, 4
  confrontational behavior in, 37
  definition of noncompliance in, 17–18

diagram on, 28, 97, 222
improvements in, 113–114, 227
parent acquiescence in, 30, 133
parent interview on, 53–54
procrastination in, 17, 29–30, 37
reinforcement in, 30, 36–38, 97
sequence of events in, 28–30
in time out procedure, 134–135, 137
training periods on, 114–115, 226
Compliant behavior, 111–119, 226
  effective commands in, 113–114, 227
  praise for, 113, 115
  in public places, 151
  in time out procedure, 137
  training periods on, 114–115, 226
Conduct disorder, 2, 4, 19
  age of onset, 26
  behavior rating scales in, 58, 59
  diagnosis of, 12, 23, 24, 44
    parent interview in, 193–195
  intervention criteria in, 20
  legal and ethical issues in, 68
  and oppositional behavior, 23–24
  prevalence of, 26
Conflict level in family, 27–30
Conners behavior rating scale, 58
Consequences of behavior
  in acquiescence, 30, 133
  as cause of misbehavior, 39, 97–98
  consistency of, 29, 36, 39, 82
    in time out procedure, 133, 142
  immediacy of, 81, 135
  reinforcement in. *See* Reinforcement
  specificity of, 82
  in time out procedure, 133, 135
Consistency of responses, 29, 36, 39, 82
  in time out procedure, 133, 142
Contextual factors, 41–42
Cost considerations, 183
  in assessment procedures, 46, 56
  breakage fees in, 75–76, 78
  in clinic or home training, 74
  in group training, 74–75, 80
Criminal behavior, 69–70
Custody issues, 68

Daily school behavior report card, 86–87, 155–
    158
  advantages of, 241–242
  discontinuation of, 163
  examples of, 156–157, 242–246
  homework assignments in, 158
  implementation of, 156–158
  parent handout on, 156, 157, 240–246
  token system in, 86–87, 157–158
Delinquent behavior, 70
Demographic information, 48, 170

Depression
  in child, 202–205
  in parent, 9, 40, 65–66, 70
Destructive behavior, 19, 45
Development
  appropriate for program, 2–3
  as cause of misbehavior, 96
  form on history of, 46, 171–173
  milestones in, 172–173
  parent interview on, 48–49, 184, 190, 191
  persistence of behavior in, 32–33
  prediction of outcome in, 33–34
Diagnosis
  in child, 8, 12, 70–71
    appropriate for program, 2
    and degree of noncompliance, 22–26
    and outcome of program, 4–5
    parent interview in, 49–54, 192–207
  in parent, 9
Discipline, 86
  consistency in, 29, 36, 39, 82
    in time out procedure, 133, 142
  and incentive programs, 82–83, 84–85
  in public, 150, 151–152, 237–238
  response cost in, 4, 132–133, 143
  spanking in, 12–13
  time out in. See Time out procedure
  in token systems, 127, 132–133
Disruptive behavior, 18–19
  diagnosis of disorder, 195
  parent attention to, 116
Disruptive Behavior Disorders Rating Scale,
    46, 47, 58
  in follow-up, 163, 164
  parent form, 59, 174–175
  in reassessment, 92, 121, 148
  teacher form, 47, 176
Distress, in intervention criteria, 21
Drug therapy in ADHD, 163–164
Dysthymic disorder, 202–203

Education level of parents, 5, 8
Effective commands, 113–114, 227
Emotional problems, 39, 94, 191
Empathy of therapist for parents, 79
Ethical issues, 68–70
Ethnic factors
  in assessment, 45, 49–50, 192
  in success of program, 8, 9

Family
  conflict levels in, 27–30
  impact of noncompliant behavior in, 27–30,
    31–32
  information form on, 46, 170
  inventory on problems in, 99, 101, 220
  parent interview on, 48, 49, 185, 189, 210–
    212
  reciprocal interactions in, 83–84
  screening of, 70–72
  self-reports on problems in, 99, 179–180,
    185, 220
  stress in, 10, 41, 98–99, 220
    assessment of, 66–67
Follow-up meetings, 87, 162–164
Future behavior problems, 159–161, 247

Gender differences, 26, 50, 51
Generalization of treatment gains, 6–7
Goals of program, 3–4
Group training, 71–72, 74–75
  on attending skills, 109
  scheduling of sessions for, 79–80
  sequence of activities in, 87, 88

Handouts for parents, 215–247
  on characteristics profile, 94–97, 219
  on compliant behavior, 113, 116–117,
    226
  on daily school behavior report card, 156,
    157, 240–246
  on effective commands, 113–114, 227
  on family problems inventory, 99, 101,
    220
  on future behavior problems, 160, 247
  on good play behavior, 105–108, 223–225
  on independent play, 116–117, 228–229
  on preparation for child's evaluation, 47,
    179–187
  on public behavior, 149–152, 237–239
  on time out procedure, 134, 233–236
  on token systems, 124, 230–232
Health history, 49, 173
Home
  safety of, 101
  token systems in. See Token systems
  training program in, 74
Home Situations Questionnaire, 46, 53–54,
    59–60
  in follow-up, 163, 164
  form for, 177
  in reassessment, 92, 121, 148
Homework assignments, 71–72
  on attending skills, 110, 119
  on causes of misbehavior, 101
  compliance with, 71, 75–76
  on daily school behavior, 158
  on future behavior problems, 161
  on public behavior, 154
  review of, 87
  on time out procedure, 144, 146
  on token systems, 130
Hypothetical behavior problems, 161

Immediacy of parent response, 81, 135
Incentives. See Rewards and incentives
Indications for treatment, 20–22
Indiscriminate parenting, 36
Individual training, 71–72, 74–75
  scheduling of sessions for, 79–80
  sequence of activities in, 87–88
Infant health and temperament, 172
Insurance reimbursements, 11, 46, 183
  for clinic or home-based training, 74
Interviews, 47–57, 167
  with child, 54–56, 185–186
  pamphlet on preparation for, 181–187
  with parents, 12, 47–54, 181–185
    on development, 48–49, 184, 190, 191
    on family, 48, 49, 185, 189, 210–212
    form used in, 48, 188–212
    format for, 54
    on home and public behavior, 53–54
    on major concerns, 48, 183–184, 189–
      191
    on management methods, 208
    objectives of, 182
    on positive characteristics, 53, 184, 210
    on psychiatric symptoms, 49–54, 192–
      207
    on school history, 49, 156, 184–185,
      190, 192, 209
    on treatment history, 49, 208–209
  with teachers, 52, 56–57, 186–187
Irritability of child, 39, 94–95

Language development, 48, 96, 173, 191
  appropriate for program, 2–3
Learning ability, teacher reports on, 57

Legal issues, 48, 68–70
  disclosure to parents on, 188–189

Maintenance of treatment gains, 6, 87
Manic episodes, 45, 205–207
Marital relationship
  affecting success of program, 5, 8, 70
  assessment of, 53, 64–65
  as factor in noncompliance, 41
Medical history, 46, 49, 171–173
Modeling
  of attending skills, 109, 117
  of time out procedure, 143–144
Monitoring of child, 35–36, 39, 118–119
  daily school report card in, 156
Motivation, 85
  of parents, 100–101
    breakage fees in, 75–76, 78
  rewards and incentives in. See Rewards and
    incentives

Noncompliant behavior
  definition of, 17–19
  degrees of, 22–26
  of parents, 75–76
  prevalence of, 26
Normative Adaptive Behavior Checklist, 46,
  61

Obsessive–compulsive disorders, 207
Oppositional behavior, 18–19
  four-factor model of, 39–42
  frequency of referrals for, 27
Oppositional defiant disorder, 2, 4
  behavior rating scales in, 58, 59, 60
  child interview in, 55
  conduct disorder in, 23–24
  developmental outcome in, 33–34
  diagnosis of, 12, 44, 45, 50–51
    criteria in, 22–23, 50–51, 192–193
  duration of symptoms in, 50–51
  frequency of referrals for, 27
  intervention criteria in, 20
  legal and ethical issues in, 68, 69
  in parent, 63–64
  parent interview in, 48, 49, 50–51, 192–
    193
  peer relationships in, 62
  prevalence of, 26
Outcomes in program
  expectations on, 4–6
  factors affecting, 7–11, 70
  generalization across settings, 6–7
  maintenance of, 6, 87

Pamphlet for parents, 179–187
Parents
  affecting success of program, 8–10
  attention to child. See Attention of parent
  deviant interactions with child, 34–39
  effectiveness of commands, 4, 113–114, 227
  group training of. See Group training
  handouts for. See Handouts for parents
  interviews with. See Interviews, with parents
  maintenance of treatment gains, 6, 87
  major concerns of, 179–180
    interview on, 48, 183–184, 189–191
  marital relationship of. See Marital
    relationship
  noncompliance of, 75–76
  preparation for program, 47, 179–187
    forms completed in, 46–47, 169–175
  profile of characteristics, 96, 219
  psychiatric disorders in, 9–10, 63–64

Parents (*continued*)
rating behavior of child, 57–60, 174–175
satisfaction with program, 5, 74
screening for program, 70–72
self-reports of. *See* Self-reports, of parents
single, 73–74
social isolation of, 9, 41, 53, 70
Peers
distress of, 21
relationship with, 62
Personality Inventory for Children, 58
Pervasive developmental disorder, atypical, 2, 4
Phobias, 197–199
Physical characteristics of child, 95–96
Play behavior
attention of parent to, 104–110
extended to compliant behavior, 113
handouts on, 105–108, 223–225, 228–229
in independent play, 116–118, 228–229
in narration exercise, 106
practicing of, 108–110, 117
reaction of parents in, 107–108, 112, 117–118
review of, 112–113
signs of positive feedback and approval in, 106–107, 224–225
independent, 4, 85, 116–118, 228–229
in token system, 128
Point systems, 85–86, 120–130, 230–232. *See also* Token systems
Poker chip system, 85–86, 120–130, 230–232. *See also* Token systems
Praise for behavior, 29, 35, 85
in compliance, 113, 115
in independent play, 117, 118
in public places, 151
Pregnancy, history of, 171–172
Prevention measures, 4
anticipation of problems in. *See* Anticipation of problems
Prosthetic social environment, 100, 122, 129
Psychological status
of child, 44–45
as cause of misbehavior, 39–40, 93–96
parent interview on, 49–54, 192–207
of parent, 62–67
affecting success of program, 9, 70
as factor in noncompliance, 40–41
Psychotic disorders, 207
Public settings, 35, 147–154
anticipation of problems in, 83, 86, 147–154
parent handout on, 149–152, 237–239
discipline in, 150, 151–152, 237–238
embarrassment of parents in, 152–153
homework assignments on, 154
incentives for compliance in, 150, 237
planned activities in, 150, 151, 238
think aloud–think ahead approach to, 149–150
time out procedure in, 78–79, 142, 143, 151–152, 239
Punishment. *See* Discipline

Questionnaires and forms, 165–214
on child and family information, 170
on developmental and medical history, 171–173

Disruptive Behavior Disorders Rating Scales, 174–176
general instructions for, 46, 167–168, 169
Home Situations Questionnaire, 177
in parent interview, 188–212
in preparation for first appointment, 46–47, 169–173
School Situations Questionnaire, 178
Referrals to clinic
complaints leading to, 27, 47, 48
initial assessment in, 46
Reinforcement
of appropriate behavior, 29, 35, 36, 97
in command–compliance sequence, 30, 36–38, 97
in deviant parent–child interactions, 35, 36–38
inadvertent, 34–35
intermittent, 98
negative, 30, 36–38, 97
positive, 29, 30, 35, 97
Reliability
of behavior rating scales, 57
of child interviews, 55–56, 186
of parent interviews, 47
Report card on school behavior. *See* Daily school behavior report card
Response cost procedure, 4, 143
implementation of, 132–133
Rewards and incentives, 82–83, 85
and discipline, 82–83, 84–85
for independent play, 117, 118
need for, 121–123
for parent compliance, 75–76, 78
in public places, 150, 151, 237
for school behavior, 86–87, 156, 157–158
tokens in. *See* Token systems
Role playing
on attending skills, 109
on time out procedure, 143–144

Safety considerations in home, 101
Scheduling of training sessions, 79–80
School behavior
daily report card on. *See* Daily school behavior report card
generalization of treatment to, 6–7
improving performance in, 86–87
parent interview on, 49, 156, 184–185, 190, 192, 209
prior to first appointment, 46, 47
questionnaires and forms on, 47, 57–60, 176, 178
and special education services, 45, 69
teacher interviews on, 52, 56–57, 186–187
School Situations Questionnaire, 47, 59–60, 178
Screening of family, 70–72
Self-reports, 21
of children, 60–61
in interviews, 54–56, 186
of parents, 62–67
on characteristics, 96–97, 219
on childhood behavior, 214
on current behavior, 213
Separation anxiety disorder, 199–201
Shaping procedure, 117
Siblings, 31
interview with, 182
Single parents, 73–74

Situational pervasiveness, 31
assessment of, 46, 59
Social behavior, 94, 192
Social ecology of family, 31–32
Social isolation of parents, 9, 41, 70
assessment of, 53
Social phobia, 198–199
Socioeconomic factors
in government entitlements, 69
in noncompliant behavior, 41
in success of program, 8, 9, 70
Socratic style of therapists, 76–77, 161
Spanking of children, 12–13
Special time period with child
establishment of, 104–110, 223–225
review of, 112
Stress
as cause of misbehavior, 41, 98–99
of parent, 10, 66–67

Teacher reports, 156, 167
behavior rating scales in, 47, 57–60, 176
in daily report card, 157, 158, 240–246
in interviews, 52, 56–57, 186–187
prior to family evaluation, 46, 47
Temperament
of child, 39–40, 93–95
history of, 172
parent handout on, 94–95, 219
of parent, 40–41, 96–97, 219
Therapist
characteristics affecting success of program, 10–11, 76–79
Socratic style of, 76–77, 161
Think aloud–think ahead method
in public places, 149–150
in transition activities, 153–154
Time out procedure, 4, 85, 86, 131–146
with aggressive children, 141
consistency in, 133, 142
duration of, 135–137, 142, 234
escape from, 12–13, 137–141, 234–235
extended to other behavior, 145–146
homework assignments on, 144, 146
location of chair in, 135, 235
modeling of, 143–144
parent handout on, 134, 233–236
preparation for, 133–134
in public, 78–79, 142, 143, 151–152, 239
reaction of parents to, 133, 141–142
restrictions in first week, 142–143, 235
Token systems, 85–86, 120–130, 230–232
advantages of, 123–124
discontinuation of, 163
establishment of, 124–127
precautions in, 127–129
homework assignments on, 130
minimum period of use, 130
need for, 121–123, 129–130
parent handout on, 124, 230–232
in public places, 150, 151, 237, 238
reaction of parents to, 129–130
response cost in, 132–133, 143
for school behavior, 86–87, 157–158
time out procedure in, 86
Tourette's disorder, 49, 207

Vineland Adaptive Behavior Scale, 46, 61
Violent behavior, 45, 141